Interp...

CHEST X-RAY

Interpretation of
CHEST X-RAY
An Illustrated Companion

G Balachandran MD DNB DMRD
Associate Professor
Department of Radiology
Sri Manakula Vinayakar Medical College and Hospital
Puducherry, India

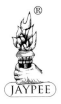

JAYPEE BROTHERS MEDICAL PUBLISHERS (P) LTD

New Delhi • London • Philadelphia • Panama

Jaypee Brothers Medical Publishers (P) Ltd

Headquarters

Jaypee Brothers Medical Publishers (P) Ltd
4838/24, Ansari Road, Daryaganj
New Delhi 110 002, India
Phone: +91-11-43574357
Fax: +91-11-43574314
Email: jaypee@jaypeebrothers.com

Overseas Offices

J.P. Medical Ltd
83 Victoria Street, London
SW1H 0HW (UK)
Phone: +44-2031708910
Fax: +02-03-0086180
Email: info@jpmedpub.com

Jaypee Medical Inc
The Bourse
111 South Independence Mall East
Suite 835, Philadelphia, PA 19106, USA
Phone: +1 267-519-9789
Email: jpmed.us@gmail.com

Jaypee Brothers Medical Publishers (P) Ltd
Bhotahity, Kathmandu, Nepal
Phone: +977-9741283608
Email: kathmandu@jaypeebrothers.com

Jaypee-Highlights Medical Publishers Inc
City of Knowledge, Bld. 237, Clayton
Panama City, Panama
Phone: +1 507-301-0496
Fax: +1 507-301-0499
Email: cservice@jphmedical.com

Jaypee Brothers Medical Publishers (P) Ltd
17/1-B Babar Road, Block-B, Shaymali
Mohammadpur, Dhaka-1207
Bangladesh
Mobile: +08801912003485
Email: jaypeedhaka@gmail.com

Website: www.jaypeebrothers.com
Website: www.jaypeedigital.com

Inquiries for bulk sales may be solicited at: jaypee@jaypeebrothers.com

Interpretation of Chest X-ray: An Illustrated Companion

First Edition: 2014
ISBN 978-93-5152-172-3
Printed at : Samrat Offset Pvt. Ltd.

Preface

This book is meant for all those doctors who want to gain an inside knowledge about how X-rays are interpreted. The book is written in simple medical language so that even medical students would be able to understand the principles of chest X-ray interpretation. There has never been an Indian radiology book devoted exclusively to the principles of chest X-ray interpretation and, meant for medical students. The unique feature of this book is that almost all chest X-rays are accompanied by corresponding line diagrams, some in color, in order to make the salient findings easy to understand. This book contains over 100 chest X-rays and similar number of line diagrams. The book is lavishly studded with tables to enhance the knowledge of the reader. Every effort has been made to ensure that only common diseases are dealt with. I hope and trust that this book will cater to the needs of all medical (MBBS) students belonging to all the Indian medical universities. The postgraduate medical students like MD general medicine and residents in radiology will also find this book very useful.

G Balachandran

Contents

1. Introduction   **1**
General Introduction   1
Basic Radiography   2
Basic Principles of Chest X-ray Interpretation   9

2. Normal Chest X-Ray   **12**
Normal Structures Seen in Chest X-ray—A Brief Description   12
Introduction   12
The Lungs and Fissures   12
Some Useful Signs in Chest X-ray Interpretation   22

3. Lung Opacity and Lung Lucency   **29**
Lung Opacity   29
Introduction   29
Unilateral Lung Opacity   30
Lobar Collapse Series   37
Collapse/Atelectasis   37
Collapse of Individual Lobes   43
Hilum Based Opacity   57
Bilateral Lung Opacity   60
Lung Lucency   64
Lung Lucency—Unilateral Involving Whole Lung   64
Lung Lucency—Unilateral Involving Part of Lung   65
Bullous Emphysema   70
Bronchiectasis   70
Lung Lucency—Bilateral COPD   72

4. Diseases of the Heart   **75**
Criteria for a Normal Heart in Chest X-ray   75
Method of Measuring CTR in Chest X-ray   76
How to Read X-ray Chest in Cardiology?   79
Cardiac Shape—A Guide to Congenital Heart Disease   84
Cardiac Situs—A Guide to CHD   87
Coarctation of Aorta   88
Patent Ductus Arteriosus (PDA)   89
Ventricular Septal Defect (VSD)   90
Atrial Septal Defect (ASD)   91
Primary Pulmonary Hypertension   92
Bicuspid Aortic Valve   93
Mitral Regurgitation   95
Rheumatic Mitral Stenosis   96
Left Atrial Enlargement   98

Pericardial Effusion   98
Calcific Pericarditis   99
Dilated Cardiomyopathy   100
Congestive Heart Failure—CHF/CCF   101
Pulmonary Edema   102
Aortic Aneurysm   103

5.   Miscellaneous Lesions   **105**
Rib Fracture   105
Cervical Rib   106
Complete Eventration of the Right Hemidiaphragm   106
Diaphragm Rupture   108
Diaphragmatic Hernia in a Child   110
Gas Under Diaphragm   111
Chilaiditi Syndrome   112

Index   ***117***

Introduction

Chapter Outline

❑ General Introduction
❑ Basic Radiography

❑ Basic Principles of Chest X-ray Interpretation

❑ GENERAL INTRODUCTION

There are no great textbooks for young doctors, medical students (and, for that matter, interns) who want to learn the basics of chest film interpretation. Radiology is not a part of curriculum, even at medical postgraduate level. Nobody is there to teach radiology to budding doctors. Most of the doctors just have a bird's eye view during the rounds. As medical students and interns you will be caring for a great number of patients on whom you will be ordering chest X-rays. While most films will ultimately be interpreted by a radiologist, you will nevertheless be expected to look at any film you order and you should have some comfort in making general diagnoses in these films without having to wait for the "official read". Many chest films are obtained even at night, both in the Emergency Department and in the hospital. These films may have abnormalities that are immediately life-threatening (e.g. Tension pneumothorax). Your responsibility is to the patient, and the sooner you can make the diagnosis, the better of the patient will be.

The goal of this book, therefore, is to attempt to simplify the process of looking at and interpreting chest films. I will ignore some of the technical jargon and subtle details in the interest of compacting the information into an easily-digested format. In addition, I will focus primarily on those findings which you may encounter at night or as an emeregency or when a radiologist may not be available to you, and on those findings which are particularly time sensitive. Only cases which are important in day-to-day practice, of a young doctor, is included.

Chest X-ray (CXR) is one which any medical doctor would come across in his day-to-day practice, irrespective of his speciality, designation or seniority. In casualties and emergencies, CXR have to be interpreted by duty doctors. Chest imaging is an important tool in managing critically ill-patients. In ICU chest radiographs are obtained routinely on a daily basis for every critical care patient, with the goal of effective clinical management. Such is the importance of a CXR. By learning some basic skills in interpreting and evaluating chest radiographs, junior doctors can recognize and localize gross pathologic changes visible on a chest radiograph. Sometimes X-rays have to be interpreted, in life-threatening situations, in which immediate decision have to be taken. Traditionally, GPs rarely see and interpret X-rays. Learning to interpret X-rays is a skill learned as a junior hospital doctor that should not be lost. There may be occasions when a GP has to make decisions based on an unreported film.

❑ BASIC RADIOGRAPHY

X-rays have very short wavelengths of electromagnetic radiation that penetrate matter. A traditional radiograph is created when X-rays penetrate body structure and produce images on a piece of photographic film usually contained in a cassette. However, in most hospitals and medical centers, the traditional X-ray film has been replaced with digital images. The basics of chest X-ray interpretation is the same irrespective of whether it is a digital image or conventional X-ray film.

Black and White Principles

- White color indicates lack of exposure and black color indicates intense exposure.
- Dense substances absorb all the rays and appear white on the film – radiopaque.
- Soft tissues and air absorb part of the beam and appear gray (tissues) or black (air) – radiolucent.

Basic Chest X-ray Views

A chest X-ray is a 2D projection of a 3D thoracic viscera. Therefore, what we see in a chest X-ray is a summated and compressed image.

Two of the most common chest radiographs are posteroanterior (PA) and anteroposterior (AP), both taken in frontal projections.

For PA views (Fig. 1.1), the X-ray beam passes through the chest from the back to the front.

For AP views (Fig. 1.2), the beam passes through the chest from the front to the back.

By convention most of the PA views are taken with patient in erect posture and most of the AP views are taken with patient in supine posture. For acutely ill patients who are bedridden and who cannot stand up for a PA view, AP views are obtained with a portable X-ray machine.

Posteroanterior (PA) View vs Anteroposterior (AP) View

There are certain findings that can distinguish a supine AP from erect PA view (Table 1.1). For e.g. PA view shows the scapulae clear of the lungs whilst in AP view they always overlap. The clavicles are overlie the lung fields in PA view, while in AP they are usually projected above the lung apices. The level of the diaphragm is lowest in PA view, while in AP view they are placed higher up. Further the heart looks bigger on an AP view because of the technical magnification In an erect film, the gastric air bubble is clearly seen in the fundus with a clear fluid level just below the left dome of diaphragm. In a supine film, blood will flow more to the apices of the

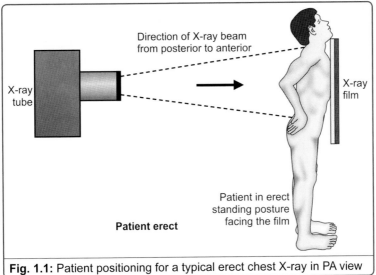

Fig. 1.1: Patient positioning for a typical erect chest X-ray in PA view

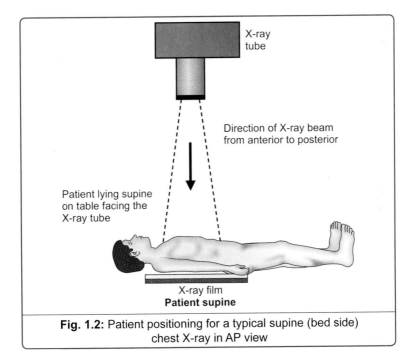

Fig. 1.2: Patient positioning for a typical supine (bed side) chest X-ray in AP view

lungs than when erect. Failure to appreciate this will lead to a misdiagnosis of pulmonary congestion. The recognising a chest X-ray film as AP or PA view is of very important as the normal anatomy significantly changes (Fig. 1.3). Therefore, doctors have to be careful about this aspect before interpreting any abnormality.

Table 1.1 PA view and AP view in chest X-ray—a comparison

	Parameter	PA view (Posteroanterior)	AP view (Anteroposterior)
1.	Patient posture	Erect (standing)	Supine (lying on back)
2.	Scapulae	Away from lung fields	Ovelie lung fields
3.	Clavicle	Project over lung zones	Project above lung apices
4.	Distinct ribs end	Posterior end	Anterior end
5.	Patients hands	Placed on hips	On the sides of thorax
6.	Heart magnification	Minimal, negligible	Moderate, significant
7.	Cardiothoracic ratio	Normal 1:2	Spuriously increased
8.	Diaphragm	Lowest level	Highest level
9.	Gastric air/fluid	Seen	Not seen, only gas seen
10.	Respiratory phase	Deep inspiration	Mid inspiration or expiration
11.	Lung expansion	Maximal	Restricted
12.	Lung markings	Normal, only lower zone vessels prominent due to gravity	Crowded, upper zone vessels unduly prominent
13.	Lung volume	Normal	Apparently reduced

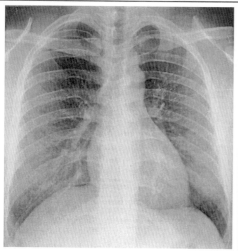
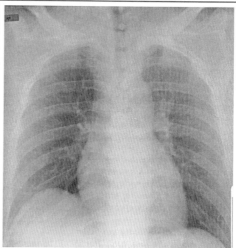

Chest PA view erect
Note the low diaphragm
Air-fluid level in stomach
Narrow superior mediastinum
Normal cardiac silhouette
Scapula away from lung zones

Chest AP view supine
Note the highly placed diaphragm
No air-fluid level in stomach
Widened superior mediastinum
Enlarged cardiac silhouette
Scapula over lung zones

Fig. 1.3: Chest X-ray for demonstrating effects of various patient positioning

Technical Factors of Viewing for Chest Radiographs

It is necessary to consider whether each of the following radiographic factors are adequate or appropriate for proper assessment of chest radiograph findings.

Penetration

X-rays must adequately penetrate body parts to visualize the structures. Ideally, one should be able to faintly see the thoracic spine, beyond fourth thoracic level, through the heart shadow, if proper penetration is employed. There are two types of improper penetration—underpenetration and overpenetration.

If you cannot clearly visualize the structures (as if it is fogged) in the chest X-ray then the radiograph is *underpenetrated* or too light (Fig. 1.4A). A poorly penetrated film looks diffusely bright and soft tissue structures are readily obscured, especially those behind the heart. In addition, the pulmonary markings may appear more prominent than they really are and may be interpreted as interstitial pulmonary edema or pulmonary fibrosis.

On the other hand if all thoracic vertebrae are seen, it is *overpenetrated*, too dark. The lung markings may appear to be absent or decreased. It is then impossible to make the judgment that

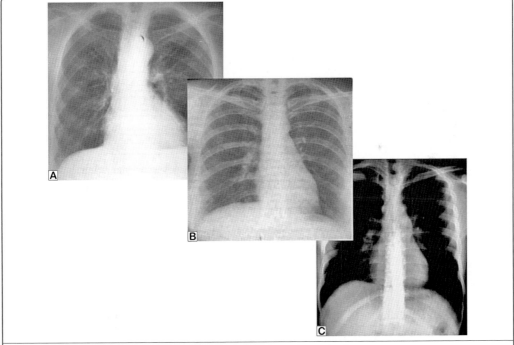

Figs 1.4A to C: Chest X-ray showing differerent types of penetration
(A) Underexposure, "Too white" all vertebral bodies, not visible chances of misdiagnosis
(B) Optimal exposure, vertebral bodies just visible through the heart
(C) Overexposure, "Too dark" all vertebral bodies seen, chances of misdiagnosis

the patient has emphysema or pneumothorax. One could also miss a pulmonary nodule when the chest radiograph is overpenetrated. An overpenetrated film looks diffusely dark and features such as lung markings are poorly seen (Fig. 1.4C).

Both under and overpenetrated X-ray film not good for reporting.

Figure 1.4B shows optimal penetration. These man made errors of X-ray technique are largely overcome by modern day computerized radiography (CR). Further in modern day CR no film processing in a dark room is done. It is a filmless and dry technique.

The computer can adjust the shortcoming in radiographic technique.

Respiration

Ideally CXR should be taken with the patient in full *inspiration.*

The anatomical findings changes in various phases of respiratioinare shown in Table 1.2.

A CXR in full inspiration should have the diaphragm as low as possible, atleast at the level of the sixth rib anteriorly and eighth rib posteriorly (Fig. 1.5). If one can count 10 posterior ribs above the diaphragm, it is an excellent inspiratory film.

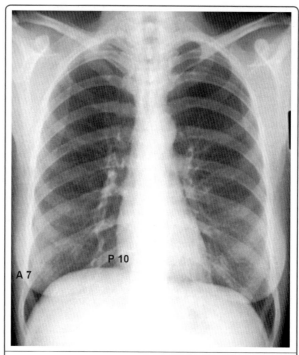

Fig. 1.5: Chest X-ray to assess depth of inspiration. The X-ray shows the right dome of diaphragm at anterior seventh rib and posterior tenth rib, indicating good respiratory effort. (Note the medical ends of clavicles are equidistant from midline indicating that the patient has not been rotated.)

Table 1.2 | Anatomical changes in chest in various respiratory phases seen normally

	Anatomical part	Inspiration	Expiration
1.	Superior mediastinum	Normal	Magnified
2.	Trachea	Straight	May be buckled
3.	Heart	Normal size	Magnified
4.	CTR	Normal	Increased
5.	Lungs	Fully expanded	Partially expanded
6.	Bronchovascular markings	Well spread out	Crowded
7.	Diaphragm	Lowest	Highest
8.	Rib cage	Anterior ends lower	Anterior and posterior ends almost same level
9.	Lung volume	Normal	Reduced

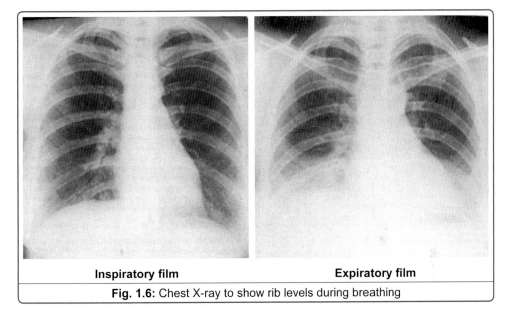

Inspiratory film	Expiratory film

Fig. 1.6: Chest X-ray to show rib levels during breathing

When less than 10 ribs can be counted above the diaphragm, it is either poor inspiratory effort or a sign of low lung volume. Low lung volume from a poor inspiration effort can crowd and compress the lung markings, producing the impression that a lower lobe pneumonia is present (Fig. 1.6).

Patient Rotation

While positioning the patient, any rotation patient is to be avoided. Ideally the patient is to positioned straight with spine in midline. It can be assessed by comparing the medial ends of the clavicles. They should be equidistant from midline as shown in Figure 1.7.

Patient rotation changes the normal thoracic anatomy, especially the mediastinum producing spurious enlargement. Rotation means that the patient was not positioned flat on the X-ray

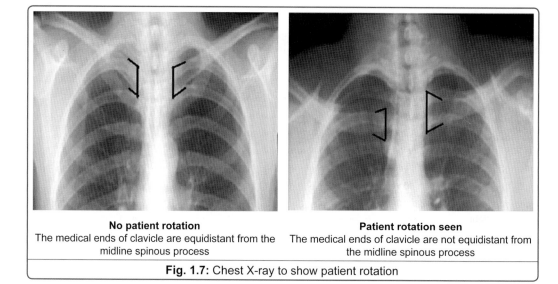

No patient rotation	**Patient rotation seen**
The medical ends of clavicle are equidistant from the midline spinous process	The medical ends of clavicle are not equidistant from the midline spinous process

Fig. 1.7: Chest X-ray to show patient rotation

film, with one plane of the chest rotated compared to the plane of the film. It causes distortion because it can make the lungs look asymmetrical and the cardiac silhouette distorted. Look for the right and left lung fields having nearly the same diameter, and the heads of the ribs (end of the calcified section of each rib) at the same location to the chest wall, which indicate absence of significant rotation. If there is significant rotation, the side that has been lifted appears narrower and denser (whiter) and the cardiac silhouette appears more in the opposite lung field.

Patient Movement

X-rays are usually taken without any movement of patient including breath holding. Movement blurring mars the image quality and loss of details.

Criteria for a technically good quality chest X-ray are shown in Table 1.3. The normal adult chest X-ray findings expected are shown in Table 1.4.

Table 1.3   Criteria for a good quality chest X-ray in adults

	Parameter	*Criteria for a good quality*	*Comments*
1.	X-ray beam direction	PA (posteroanterior)	In all ambulant patients
2.	Patient body position	Erect	Gravity helps lung expansion
3.	Patient rotation	Nil	Clavicle equidistant, spine midline
4.	Respiratory phase	Deep inspiration	Diaphragm at lowest position
5.	Depth of respiration	Diaphragm level	Eight anterior or ten posterior ribs seen
6.	Technical factors	X-ray penetration/exposure (Radiographic density)	Adequate so that the lower thoracic spine is just seen through the heart shadow
7.	Artifacts	No blurring of image	Movement artifacts mars the image quality

Table 1.4 | Normal adult chest X-ray

	Parameter	Criteria	Comments
1.	Penetration	Should be adequate	Overpenetration – too black film Underpenetration – too white film Buckled indicates expiration
2.	Trachea	Straight, in midline, spine to be seen through it	Altered in expiration/supine films
3.	Mediastinum	Only 1/3 of heart seen in right of midline side and 2/3 to the left of midline	Altered in expiration/supine films
4.	CTR	Normally 1:2	Altered in expiration/supine films
5.	Lung zones	Well aerated in fully expanded lungs	Altered in expiration/supine films
6.	Diaphragm Height Level Shape	Right dome 2–3 cm higher than left dome. Anterior 8th rib or posterior 9th rib, dome shaped	Because of heart lying on left dome Altered in expiration/supine films Altered in expiration/supine films
7.	CP angles	Sharp, acutely angled in both sides	Altered in expiration/supine films

❑ BASIC PRINCIPLES OF CHEST X-RAY INTERPRETATION

Radiographic Density

When referring to radiographic shadowing, the term 'density' refers to the radio-opacity of a lesion and this will be influenced fundamentally by the degree of exposure of the film. What we see in radiography is a measure of the optical density.

The four basic radiographic densities are (Table 1.5):

- Gas (air), which appears black or radiolucent; examples are gas or air in trachea, bronchi, or stomach
- Fat, which appears gray or less radiolucent than air; an example subcutaneous fat
- Water (soft tissue), which appears white with slight radiopacity; examples are the heart, blood vessels, muscle, and diaphragm
- Bone (or metal), which appears all white or completely radiopaque; examples are bones, ribs, clavicles, etc.

Each radiograph has a continuum of shades from black to white in its images due to the way the body structures or tissues absorb the X-ray beam. X-rays penetrate body tissues that have

Table 1.5 | Basic radiographic densities as seen in CXR

	Structures	Radiographic appearance	Examples—normal tissues	Examples—abnormal tissues
1.	Air	Dark-black (radiolucent)	Air in lungs, trachea	Surgical emphysema
2.	Fat	Gray, less dark (less radiolucent)	Fat in subcutaneous plane	Mediastinal lipomatosis
3.	Water	Fluid, light-white (less radiopaque)	Muscles, blood in heart	Pleural efusion
4.	Bone	Bright-white (radiopaque)	Clavicles, ribs	Calcific focus

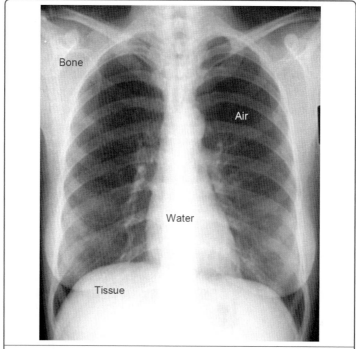

Fig. 1.8: Chest X-ray to show four basic radiographic densities

minimal tissue density, such as air or air-filled structures, and produce black or dark areas on the radiograph; these areas are referred to as *radiolucent*. Areas or body tissues that cannot be penetrated by X-rays are *radiopaque* and appear bright-white on the radiograph (Fig. 1.8).

Thus, each body tissue or structure has different radiodensity depending upon X-ray penetration.

Radiographic Contrast

If two structures of equal density [e.g. water (white) + water (white) or air (black) + air (black)] are adjacent to each other, the border of neither structure can be detected. But if two structures of different densities [e.g. water (white) + air (black)] are adjacent to each other, the border of both structure can be detected. This is because of the factor called contrast. It is the difference in the densities that is responsible for the "contrast". In normal chest X-ray the white/black difference (i.e. contrast) in optical density makes the white heart standout against the black lung (Fig. 1.9).

In the Figure 1.10 the left lung is uniformly black because the entire left lung has only air in the alveoli.

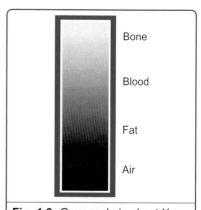

Fig. 1.9: Gray scale in chest X-ray

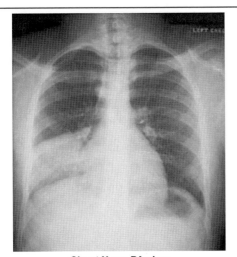

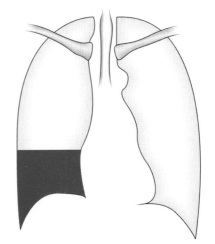

Chest X-ray PA view
The right heart border silhouetee is lost.
The right dome of diaphragm is well seen.
Therefore the lesion must be in right middle lobe.

A well defined opacity in right lower zone
The difference in the radiographic density between
right upper lobe and right middle lobe makes the
finding obvious.
The upper zone is black, while the lower zone is white.

Fig. 1.10: Chest X-ray to show the radiographic contrast

In the right side the lower zone lung has exudates in the alveoli and hence appears opaque. Because of this difference in the radiographic density one can distinguish different pathologies. Thus in the X-ray there is lung consolidation involving the middle lobe.

The normal silhouette (outline) of heart borders, diaphragm, etc. can be well seen because of the contrast that exists naturally, between the 'white' cardiac structures and "black" adjacent lung tissue. This is the natural radiographic contrast.

Normal Chest X-ray

Chapter Outline

❑ Introduction
❑ The Lungs and Fissures

❑ Some Useful Signs in Chest X-ray Interpretation

NORMAL STRUCTURES SEEN IN CHEST X-RAY—A BRIEF DESCRIPTION

❑ INTRODUCTION

In the following pages an overview of all thoracic structures is given, emphasizing only the radiological anatomy. Each important structure is shown by chest X-rays and corresponding line diagrams. Later key points for chest X-ray interpretation is given.

There are two tables, one (Table 2.1) showing the normal structures seen in chest X-ray and the normal variants in other (Table 2.2) shows common abnormalities that are seen in common lung pathologies.

❑ THE LUNGS AND FISSURES

Since most of the lung consists of air, which is essentially transparent to X-rays (radiolucent) the only structures which are visible in normal lungs are the blood vessels, the interlobar fissures and the walls of some larger bronchi seen end on. Thus, the lungs are radiolucent, in both sides with traces of gray linear marking which are blood vessels (Fig. 2.1).

The right lung is divided into three lobes by means of two fissures: oblique and horizontal.

The oblique fissure runs from a position anterior on the diaphragm in a posterior direction superiorly towards the apex of the lung around thoracic vertebra T4 posterior, splitting the lung into an anterior, superior section (the upper and middle lobes) and a posterior, inferior section (the lower lobe). It is better seen in lateral projection.

The horizontal fissure runs from the anterior wall of the lung to the hilum, horizontally, dividing the upper section of the right lung into an upper lobe and a middle lobe. On the PA

Table 2.1 | Normal finding and normal variants (some examples)

Structure	Normal finding	Normal variants
Trachea	Central, midline, cervical spinous processes seen through the tracheal air column	Displaced to right by unfolded aorta
Heart	Normal CTR = 0.5 2/3 of heart lies to the left of midline 1/3 of heart lies to the right of midline	1. Assessment of heart size 　Difficult in AP view, obese persons 2. Geometric enlargement on AP 3. Apparent enlargement on expiration 4. Depressed sternum displaces heart
Hilum	Left 1cm above right, symmetrical, concave	Obscured partly by heart
Lung zones	Both sides show, symmetric Similar radiographic density	Rotation and absence of breast shadow will produce differences in density
Fissures	Horizontal fissure at 6th rib right side only Oblique fissure not seen	Accessory fissures, e.g. azygos in right side
Diaphragm	Smooth outline convex upwards Sharply defined costophrenic and cardiophrenic angles Right dome 2 cm above left, normally	Elevation of left dome is often due to stomach gas Frequent hump on right dome in the elderly Fat pad in obese people
Bone thoracic cage	Level of rib correspond to the depth of respiration, lower in inspiration and higher in expiration	Cervical rib and minor rib anomalies, like synostosis are common
Soft tissue	Breast in young and nipples in old age women seen sharply	Plaits, hair, artefacts

Table 2.2 | Abnormal chest X-ray findings (some examples)

	Structure	Normal finding	Abnormal finding—example only
1.	Trachea	Central	Pulled by collapse, fibrosis other lung volume reducing pathologies Pushed by massive pleural pathologies like effusion, pneumothorax
2.	Heart	Normal CTR = 0.5 Overall T diameter >16 cm 2/3 of heart lies left of midline	Increased CTR, e.g. Endocardial pathology VHD Myocardial pathology DCM Pericardial pathology effusion
3.	Hilum	Left 1 cm above right	Pulled by fibrosis, collapse Enlarged by lymphadenopathy
4.	Lung fields	Similar radiographic density	Increased density by mass consolidation, collapse, decreased density by air trapping, bullae, etc
5.	Fissures	Horizontal fissure at 6th rib right	Pulled by fibrosis, collapse
6.	Diaphragm	Smooth outline convex upwards Sharply define costophrenic angles Shadow at the level of 6th rib Right dome 2 cm above left	Pulled by fibrosis, collapse Abnormally elevated by paralysis, hepatomegaly, etc. Flatted by emphysema
7.	Thoracic cage	Calcification in costal cartilage is insignificant	Volume increases in COPD Volume decreases in collapse
8.	Soft tissue shadows	Breast and nipples	Air in SC plane

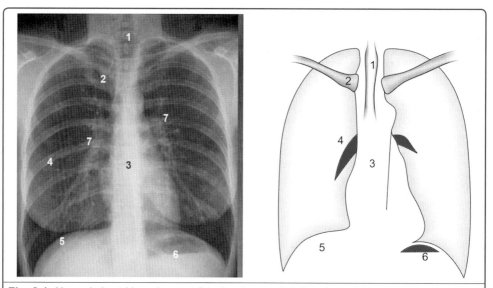

Fig. 2.1: Normal chest X-ray in erect PA view in an adult female patient

1. Trachea is straight, in midline, spinous process seen throw it, indicating no patient rotation
2. Clavicles both medial ends are equidistant from midline, indicating no patient rotation
3. Thoracic spine well seen behind the heart shadow, indicating overpenetration
4. Note the uniform blackiness in both lung zones, indicating normal aeration in both lungs
5. Note the level of diaphragm is at tenth posterior rib, indicating deep inspiration
6. Note the air/fluid level in stomach below left dome, indicating erect patient posture
7. Right and left hilum made up of normal pulmonary vessel and bronchi

film, only the horizontal fissure is visible running from the right hilum to the region of the sixth rib in the axillary line (Fig. 2.2A).

The left lung is divided into two lobes, an upper and a lower, by an oblique fissure (Fig. 2.2B) similar to the right lung. The lingula, or remnant of the middle lobe on the left, is considered to form part of the upper lobe.

The chest X-ray is a 2D projection of a 3D thoracic structures. There is considerable overlapping of lung lobes. Therefore, all the thoracic structures are summated together in a chest X-ray film. There is only a representation of all the lobes in frontal projection (Fig. 2.3). In practice the lung is divided into three zones—upper, middle and lower (Fig. 2.4) by drawing two horizontal imaginary lines—upper one passes through second rib anteriorly and the lower one through the fourth rib anteriorly, in each side. In practice the lungs are divided into zones; upper, middle, and lower zones.

• Upper; from the apex to 2nd costal cartilage
• Middle; between 2nd and 4th costal cartilage
• Lower; between 4th and 6th costal cartilage

Look for equal radiolucency (or blackness due to air filling) between the left and the right lungs zones. Look for any discrete or generalized gray/white shadows (described as opacity/patchy shadows).

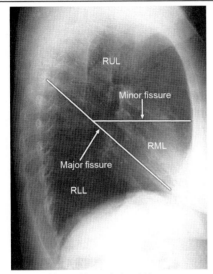

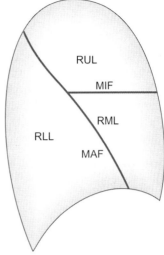

Normal lateral chest X-ray
(MIF) Minor (horizontal) fissure
(MAF) Major (oblique) fissure

The horizontal fissure runs from the anterior wall of the lung to the hilum, horizontally, dividing the upper section of the right lung into an upper lobe and a middle lobe. On the PA film, only the horizontal fissure is visible running from the right hilum to the region of the sixth rib in the axillary line.

Fig. 2.2A: Chest right lateral view to show both the fissures

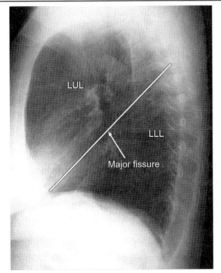

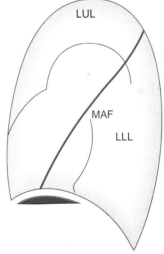

Normal lateral chest X-ray
(MAF) Major (oblique) fissure

The oblique fissure runs from a position anterior on the diaphragm in a posterior direction superiorly towards the apex of the lung around T4 posteriorly, splitting the lung into an anterior, superior section (the upper lobe) and a posterior, inferior section (the lower lobe)

Fig. 2.2B: Chest left lateral view to show oblique fissure

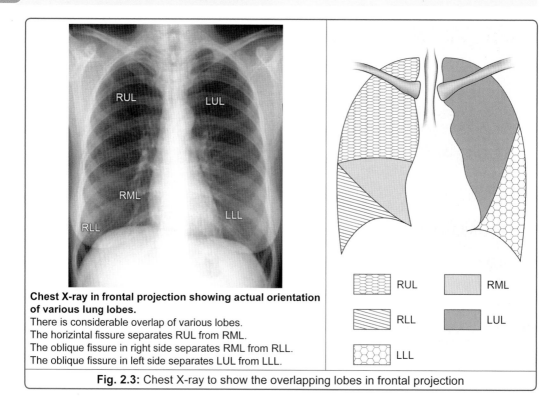

Chest X-ray in frontal projection showing actual orientation of various lung lobes.
There is considerable overlap of various lobes.
The horizintal fissure separates RUL from RML.
The oblique fissure in right side separates RML from RLL.
The oblique fissure in left side separates LUL from LLL.

Fig. 2.3: Chest X-ray to show the overlapping lobes in frontal projection

The bronchi, pulmonary artery and lymphatics form the hilum of each lung (Fig. 2.1). The left hilum is usually smaller and higher in position than the right hilum. The pulmonary arteries and veins are lighter and air is black, as it is radiolucent. Both hila should be normally concave, similar size, shape and density.

Pleural Covering

Depending upon the site enveloping the lungs the pleura is named as diaphragmatic, mediastinal, costal, and apical pleurae. There are two layers of pleura: the parietal pleura and the visceral pleura. The parietal pleura lines the thoracic cage and the visceral pleura surrounds the lung. Both of these layers come together to form reflections which separate the individual lobes. These pleural reflections are known as fissures. On the right there is an oblique and horizontal fissure; the right upperlobe sits above the horizontal fissure (HF), the right lower lobe behind the oblique fissure (OF) and the middle lobe between the two. On the left, an oblique fissure separates the upper and lower lobes.

Ribs

Both anterior (to the sternum) and posterior (to the spinal vertebrae) attachments of the ribs are visible on the chest radiograph. It is important to be clear on differentiating the two.

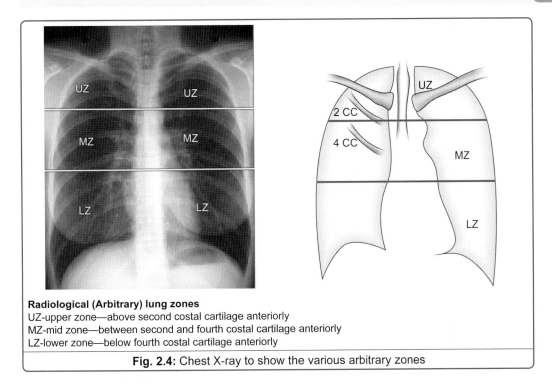

Radiological (Arbitrary) lung zones
UZ-upper zone—above second costal cartilage anteriorly
MZ-mid zone—between second and fourth costal cartilage anteriorly
LZ-lower zone—below fourth costal cartilage anteriorly

Fig. 2.4: Chest X-ray to show the various arbitrary zones

The posterior ribs lie horizontally, whereas the anterior ribs slope inferiorly joining the costochondral cartilages, which are of lower density than bone, are therefore relatively radiolucent, and so appear darker than bone (Fig. 2.5).

Diaphragm

The diaphragm is considered in two halves (left and right "hemidiaphragms") though anatomically there is only one diaphragm. Diaphragm is normally rounded and dome shaped. The right hemidiaphragm is higher than the left, on full inspiration by 2–3 cm. The pleurae near the corners of the thorax and cardiac shadow form the costophrenic and cardiophrenic recesses respectively (Fig. 2.6).

Heart

An overview of cardiac structures is shown in Figure 2.7. The heart lies in the middle mediastinum in midline. The width of the heart should be no more than half the width of the chest. This is the normal cardiothoracic ratio (CTR) (Fig. 2.8). About a third of the heart should be to the right and two thirds to the left of center. *Note:* the heart looks larger on an AP film and thus you cannot comment on the presence or absence of cardiomegaly on an AP film.
Site: Is it located on the right or left?
Size: Is it less than half the transthoracic diameter? (i.e. is the largest diameter of the heart less than half the largest diameter of the thorax)

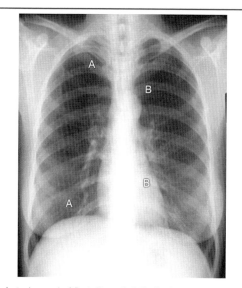

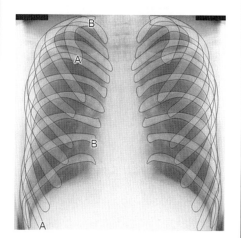

A-Anterior end of first rib and sixth rib-right side	**Bony skeleton to show rib cage**
B-Posterior end of fifth rib and ninth ribs in left side.	A-Anterior end of first rib and eighth rib-right side
Each rib has its posterior end higher up and anterior end lower down	B-Posterior end of first rib and ninth ribs in right side
Frontal view showing the oblique orientation of the ribs. The anterior portions are slanted downward and the posterior portions are slanted upward. The costal cartilages (not shown) connect the anterior ribs to the sternum	Each rib has its posterior end higher up and anterior end lower down
	C-Clavicle

Fig. 2.5: A chest X-ray—adult female—erect PA view to show orientation of ribs

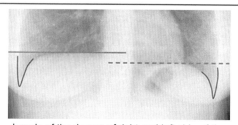

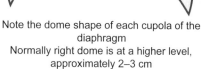

Levels of the domes of right and left side of the diaphragm	Note the dome shape of each cupola of the diaphragm
Note the sharply outlined right and left costophrenic angles	Normally right dome is at a higher level, approximately 2–3 cm

Fig. 2.6: X-ray lower chest to show the diaphragm and its recess

Shape: Is it ovoid with the apex pointing to the left?
Shadows: Any change in density?
Borders: Is it clear or well-defined?

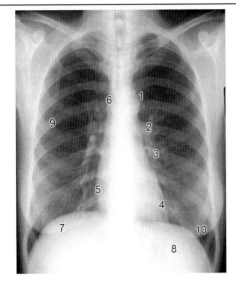
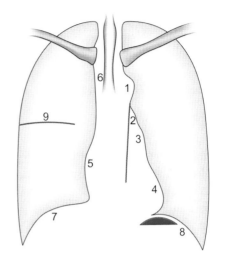

1. Aortic arch
2. Pulmonary trunk
3. Left atrial appendage
4. Left ventricle
5. Right atrium
6. Superior vena cava

7. Right hemidiaphragm
8. Left hemidiaphragm
    (note gastric air/fluid level)
9. Horizontal fissure
10. Left breast shadow.

Fig. 2.7: Normal chest X-ray in erect PA view in an adult female patient to show cardiac structures

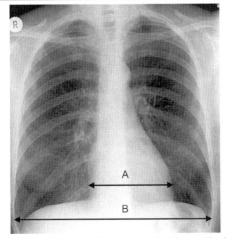
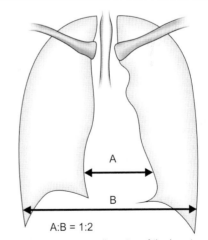

Chest X-ray in erect PA view showing the method of measuring the cardiothoracic ratio (CTR)

A. Maximum transverse diameter of the heart
B. Maximum transverse diameter of the chest
Normally the CTR (A/B) is 1:2

A:B = 1:2

Fig. 2.8: Chest X-ray to show CTR measurement

The right border is only the right atrium alone and above it is the border of the superior vena cava (Fig. 2.9). The right ventricle is anterior and so does not have a border on the PA chest X-ray film. The left atrium is the posterior most chamber and not normally seen in PA chest X-ray filmThe left border of the heart is formed by (from above downwards) aortic knob, pulmonary artery, left atrial appendage and thin strip of left ventricle (Fig. 2.10).

Key Points for Interpretation

Trachea/Bronchi/Alveoli

a. Is the trachea in midline or deviated
b. Carina (where trachea divides into right and left bronchus) should be visible with slightly blacker outline over the lung fields themselves.
   Check the carinal angle. Normally it is acute.
c. Hila: Pulmonary arteries and veins. Left hilum appears smaller and higher than the right hilum
d. Check expansion of lungs, see all the lobes, both lungs should be symmetrically black.
   Is there are any opacity—linear/segmental/mass-like, etc. Is there any air bronchogram?
e. Look for the fissures—horizontal, oblique, their course, any shift.

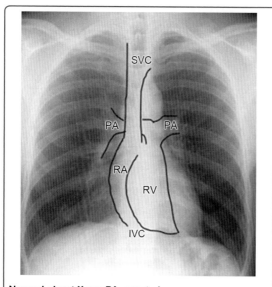

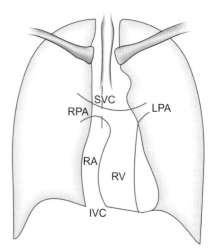

Normal chest X-ray PA, erect view
To show right heart border, position of RA, RV, PA in frontal projection

SVC-Superior vena cava
RPA-right pulmonary artery
LPA-left pulmonary artery
RA-right atrium
RV-right ventricle
IVC-inferior vena cava

Fig. 2.9: Chest X-ray with right heart structures lined out

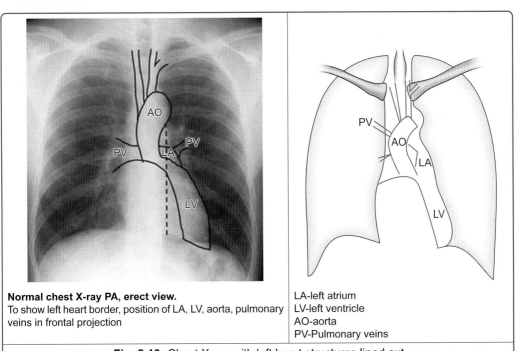

Normal chest X-ray PA, erect view.
To show left heart border, position of LA, LV, aorta, pulmonary veins in frontal projection

LA-left atrium
LV-left ventricle
AO-aorta
PV-Pulmonary veins

Fig. 2.10: Chest X-ray with left heart structures lined out

Heart and Great Vessels

a. Check size—CTR, cardiac apex.
b. Look at the cardiac site, shape, size, borders.
c. Look for any specific chamber enlargement.
d. Unclear right border suggest middle lobe consolidation.
e. Unclear left border suggest lingular lobe consolidation.
f. Check aortic arch, pulmonary artery for size, site, shape.
g. Check the pulmonary vascularity, is it increased/decreased; is it arterial/venous. Are they pruned?

Mediastinum

a. Check for mediastina size, shifts, density.
b. Check for borders—any mass/abnormal increase of structutes.

Diaphragm

a. Look for the level, shape, any tenting, flattening.
b. Look for sharp costophrenic and cardiophrenic recesses, whiteness immediately above the diaphragm indicates pleural effusion or consolidation. The presence of fluid will produce a meniscus (Meniscus sign) or a concave upper border.

c. Is the diaphragm below the anterior end of the 6th rib on the right? If so, this indicates hyperinflation.

d. Normal diaphragm elevations occur with obesity, pregnancy, pain, bowel obstruction.

e. Flatten diaphragms are indicative of emphysema.

f. Unilateral diaphragm changes are indicative of abdominal organ distention or paralysis.

g. Check sub-diaphragmatic region for abnormal air collection.

Bone Structures

a. Shape of the thorax – emphysema, polio, scoliosis?

b. Is the entire thorax visible? 9–10 posterior ribs should be visible in deep inspiration.

c. Look at and compare the bony structures paying attention to site, size, shape, shadows and borders: (clavicles, ribs, scapulae, thoracic vertebrae, and humerrus).

d. Any rib fractures? Erosion/notching/callus formation, altered density—osteoporosis, osteosclerosis.

e. Signs of surgery—rib resection, any extra rib.

f. Midline sternotomy sutures.

g. Intercostal spaces: Width and angle, wide or narrow?

Soft Tissues

a. Check neck and axilla for surgical emphysema, hemotomas, tumors.

b. Large breast tissue may obscure lung field to some extent, any e/o mastectomy.

Others

Look for any tubes (drainage, endotracheal, etc), pacemakers, catheters, artificial valve, etc.

A, B, C'S of Chest X-ray Interpretation

A- Airways—trachea, bronchi, alveoli

B- Bone cage—ribs, thoracic vertebrae other bones seen—clavicle, scapula
   Blood vessels—aorta, pulmonary artery

C- Cardiac structures—CTR, chambers, borders

D- Diaphragm domes, costophrenic and cardiphrenic angles

E- Extrathoracic structures—chest wall, breast, sub-diaphragmatic, supraclavicular region

F- Fissures—oblique, horizontal

G- Gastric air bubble, great vessels—aorta, pulmonary artery

H- Hilum

❏ SOME USEFUL SIGNS IN CHEST X-RAY INTERPRETATION

Silhouette Sign

The normal silhouette (outline) of heart borders, diaphragm, etc. can be well seen because of the contrast that exists naturally between the "white" cardiac structures and "black" adjacent lung tissue.

The silhouette sign is the absence of depiction of an anatomic soft-tissue border. It is caused by consolidation and/or atelectasis of the adjacent lung, by a large mass, or by contiguous pleural fluid. The silhouette sign results from the juxtaposition of structures of similar radiographic density. The sign actually refers to the absence of a silhouette. This phenomenon, called the silhouette sign, is used not only to identify normal chest structures but also diagnose and localize lung diseases. Further the silhouette sign may be used to distinguish anterior from posterior structures on a chest radiograph.

For example, a silhouette sign would be expected in an area of consolidation in the right middle lobe of the lung because this lobe borders the right sides of the right atrium and the mediastinum. Because both the area of consolidation and the heart are water densities (white), the right border of the right atrium cannot be distinguished from the border of the right middle lobe of the lung. That is the right heart border is obscured, if the adjacent lung (right middle lobe) is consolidated (Fig. 2.11).

Uses of Silhouette Sign

1. Helps in localization of disease either in lungs or mediastinum in a chest X-ray, e.g. if a lesion is close to right heart border and obscures this right heart border, then the lesion is only in the right middle lobe of the lungs.

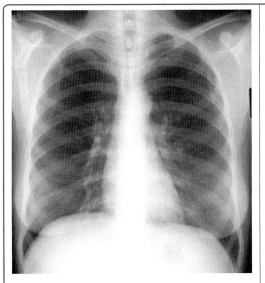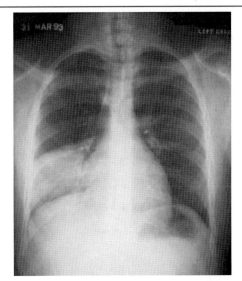

| Note the well seen right heart border in a normal female. The white right heart border is well seen with the black density in right middle lobe region. Normally the right middle lobe (RML) is adjacent to right heart margin and does not reach diaphragm. | Note the right heart border is obscured in RML consolidation. This is positive silhouette sign. The loss of right heart border silhouette has helped in localizing the lung pathology to middle lobe. Hence if the right heart margin is indistinct with a sharp diaphragm the lesion has to be in the RML. |

Fig. 2.11: Chest X-ray showing application of silhouette sign in right middle lobe consolidation

2. The silhouette sign may be used to distinguish structures in anterior plane from those in posterior plane in a chest X-ray, e.g. if a mass in left side of superior mediastinum obscures the aortic knob then the mass must be in posterior plane. In case of anteriorly placed mass the aortic knob would be seen through the mass.

3. To localize the particular lobe of involvement, e.g. an opacity in right lower zone, if it obscures the right heart border, then it must be from right middle lobe. For in right lower lobe opacities the right border is not obscured. On the other hand if the opacity obscures the right dome of diaphragm, then the lesion must be from lower lobe.

Caution: Pleural disease can obliterate all the silhouettes, e.g. right side pleural effusion will obscure all right-sided Silhouette viz right dome of diaphragm, right heart border, ascending aorta.

In order to use silhouette sign effectively one need to know the location of each silhouette and the lung tissue adjacent to it. They are shown in Figure 2.12 and Table 2.3. The loss of silhouette in various lung pathologies are shown in Table 2.4.

Air Bronchogram Signs

Branching, linear, tubular lucency representing a bronchus or bronchiole passing through airless lung parenchyma. This sign indicates that the underlying opacity must be parenchymal rather than pleural or mediastinal in location.

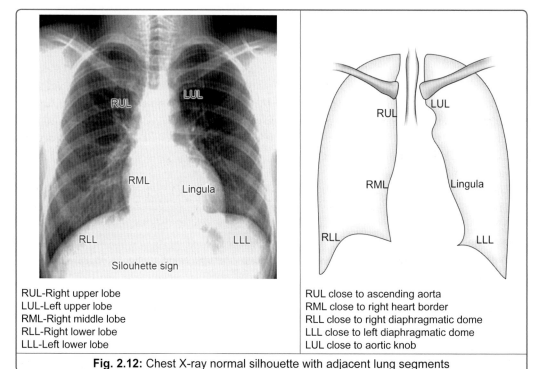

RUL-Right upper lobe	RUL close to ascending aorta
LUL-Left upper lobe	RML close to right heart border
RML-Right middle lobe	RLL close to right diaphragmatic dome
RLL-Right lower lobe	LLL close to left diaphragmatic dome
LLL-Left lower lobe	LUL close to aortic knob

Fig. 2.12: Chest X-ray normal silhouette with adjacent lung segments

Table 2.3 | Normal silhouette with adjacent lung segments

Normal silhouette	Adjacent lung structure
Right diaphragmatic dome	Right lower lobe, basal segments
Right heart margin	Right middle lobe-medial segment
Ascending aorta	RUL, anterior segment,
Aortic knob	LUL, posterior segment
Left heart margin	Lingula
Left diaphragmatic dome	Left lower lobe, basal segments
Descending aorta	LLL/superior and medial segments

Table 2.4 | Examples of application of loss of silhouette

	Silhouette lost	Adjacent pathology in	Classic e.g.
1.	Right heart border	Right middle lobe	Collapse/consolidation
2.	Left heart border	Left lingular segment	Collapse/consolidation
3.	Right dome diaphragm	Right lower lobe	Collapse/consolidation
4.	Left dome diaphragm	Left lower lobe	Collapse/consolidation
5.	Aortic knuckle	Left upper lobe	Collapse/consolidation aortic aneurysm

Differential diagnosis: Pneumonia, lymphoma, bronchoalveolar cell carcinoma (Fig. 2.13).

Normally the air that is present in the bronchial tree is taken upto the alveoli for gas exchange. If alveoli are filled with fluid (instead of air) as in consolidation, the air in the bronchial tree gets stranded. This ability to visualize distal bronchial tree as air filled, branching, dark tubular structures is called air bronchogram. This occurs when the alveoli are filled and the bronchial tree is patent. Alveolar filling displaces air with a liquid density and provides a contrast to visualize air filled bronchi.

The air (black) stands out against the fluid (white) background. Thus, the air in the bronchial tree is made visible. This is called air bronchogram and is a sure sign of alveolar pathology.

- Ability to visualize distal bronchial tree as air filled dark tubular structures is called air bronchogram.
- This occurs when the alveoli are filled with exudates replacing air and the bronchial tree is patent.

Air Bronchogram

- Alveolar filling displaces air with a liquid density and provides a contrast to visualize air filled bronchi.
- Presence of air bronchogram indicative of and a definite sign of alveolar pathological process.

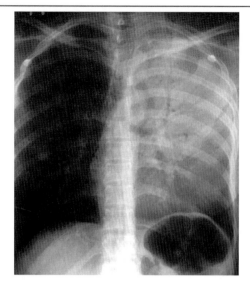
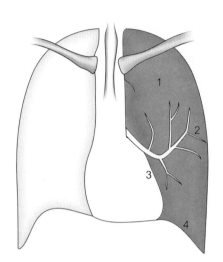

Homogenous opacity left upper and mid zones
1. Air bronchogram
2. Loss of left heart border silhouette
3. Left dome diaphragm well seen
4. No evidence of push/pull
5. Normal CP angles
6. No volume loss

No signs of push/pull
1. Homogenous opacity left side thorax
2. Classic air bronchogram
3. Loss of left heart border silhouette
4. Left diaphragm dome well seen
Consolidation left lung upper lobe including lingular segment

Fig. 2.13: Chest X-ray to show air bronchogram signs

- Consolidation is a pathological term. It describes the state of the lung when alveolar gas has been replaced by exudates (pneumonia), fluid (pulmonary odema), cells (bronchoalveolar carcinoma) or a mixture of the above. Therefore, the lesion are aptly called alveolar filling or air-space filling disease.

Causes of Air Bronchogram

Common	**Rare**
Expiratory film	Lymphoma
Consolidation	Alveolar cell carcinoma
Pulmonary oedema	Sarcoidosis
Hyaline membrane disease	Fibrosing alveolitis
Alveolar proteinosis	Radiation fibrosis
ARDS	

Tram Lines

If the bronchi are recognizable beyond 5th order of branching it is abnormal. This can occur when the bronchial walls become visible. If the bronchi wall is thickened as in chronic bronchitis,

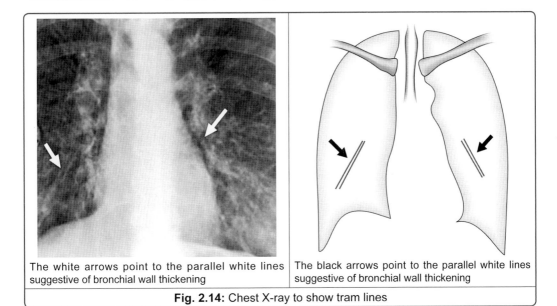

| The white arrows point to the parallel white lines suggestive of bronchial wall thickening | The black arrows point to the parallel white lines suggestive of bronchial wall thickening |

Fig. 2.14: Chest X-ray to show tram lines

bronchiectasis or there is cartilaginous calcification then one can recognize them also. The air filled bronchial lumen shows tram line appearance (Fig. 2.14). These cast parallel tram line shadows which, when seen end-on, appear as ring shadows. They are a common finding in bronchiectasis, recurrent asthma, bronchopulmonary as per gillosis pulmonary edema and lymphangitis carcinomatosis. If the peribronchial interstitial space becomes thickened by fluid or tumor, the walls are less clearly defined.

Extrapleural Sign

The extrapleural fat sign refers to the fat layer outside the pleura in the chest wall between the parietal pleura and the endothoracic fascia. Any mass located here will appear peripherally located with sharp inner margin and indistinct outer margin. The mass usually makes a concave angle with the chest wall and appears equal size in all projections (Fig. 2.15).

This sign is useful to differentiate pleural from lung/mediastinal masses.

Recognition of this finding on is useful to determine the extrapleural location of a lesion, as it is outlined by a fat ribbon that represents the extrapleural fat medially displaced. The extrapleural fat sign is the inward displacement of an extrapleural fat stripe by an extrapleural fluid collection or mass. Expanding lesions of structures in the chest wall give rise to this sign.

Explanation: Extrapleural fat, endothoracic fascia, and the innermost layers of intercostal muscle are superficial to the parietal pleura. Extrapleural fat is usually seen as a 1 mm thick and is almost imperceptible in normal individuals. It may be thicker in obese patients. Accumulation of blood in the extrapleural space results in an extrapleural hematoma (EPH), which displaces

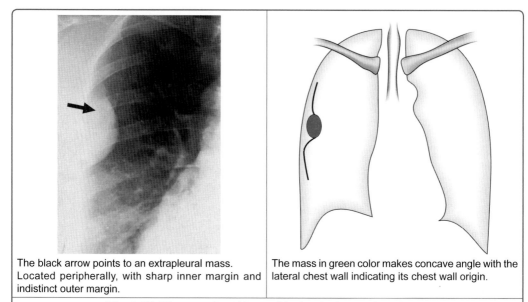

| The black arrow points to an extrapleural mass. Located peripherally, with sharp inner margin and indistinct outer margin. | The mass in green color makes concave angle with the lateral chest wall indicating its chest wall origin. |

Fig. 2.15: Shows a chest X-ray with classical extrapleural sign

the overlying extrapleural fat centrally and is most commonly the result of injury to intercostal arteries or veins. EPH is an underreported complication of blunt chest trauma.

Lung Opacity and Lung Lucency

Chapter Outline

❑ Introduction
❑ Unilateral Lung Opacity
❑ Lobar Collapse Series
❑ Collapse/Atelectasis
❑ Collapse of Individual Lobes
❑ Hilum-based Opacity

❑ Bilateral Lung Opacity
❑ Lung Lucency—Unilateral Involving Whole Lung
❑ Lung Lucency—Unilateral Involving Part of Lung
❑ Bullous Emphysema
❑ Bronchiectasis
❑ Lung Lucency–Bilateral COPD

LUNG OPACITY

❑ INTRODUCTION

In this chapter abnormal chest X-ray findings are discussed based on the predominant X-ray finding, viz. lung opacity and lung lucency. Each radiographic density is discussed further based on involvement of the particular lung—whether unilateral or bilateral; or whether it is entire lung or part of the lung that is involved. The most common cause of unilateral hemithorax opacification is due to pleural effusion. Other causes include one lung massive collapse, surgical removal, massive consolidation and post infective sequelae (Table 3.1). The X-ray finding in common conditions are described along with line diagrams in order to make the xray interpretation easy. Further brief notes on common pathologies and their radiological features are discussed in the following chapters. The causes of unilateral lung opacity is given in Table 3.1.

Table 3.1 | Causes of opacification of a hemithorax

1. Massive pleural effusion
2. Massive collapse
3. Massive consolidation
4. Pneumonectomy
5. Fibrothorax
6. Massive tumor
7. Combination of above lesions
8. Lung agenesis

❑ UNILATERAL LUNG OPACITY

Unilateral Lung Opacity Involving Whole Lung

Lung opacity involving one entire hemithorax is most commonly due to a pleural effusion.

Usually pleural effusion produces uniform homogenous opacity, unless complicated. With massive pleural effusion the signs of "push" predominate-entire mediastinum (trachea and heart) is pushed to opposite side, intercostal spaces in same side are widened. These findings are visible on a chest X-ray (Fig. 3.1). The pulmonary vessels and fissure are not seen because the lungs has already (passively) collapsed. The ipsilateral heart border and the diaphragmatic dome are obscured due to "silhouette sign" effect (Table 3.2). In cases of collapse the signs of "pull" due to loss of lung volume predominate. In massive unilateral lung collapse entire hemithorax show opacity. The "air bronchogram" may or may not be visible. But signs of pull such as mediastinal (trachea and heart) shift towards the same side as the lesion, narrowing of the same side intercostal spaces and abnormal elevation of ipsilateral diaphragmatic dome are seen well in a chest X-ray (Fig. 3.2). The pulmonary vessels and fissure are not seen because the lungs has already (actively) collapsed. The ipsilateral heart border and the diaphragmatic dome are obscured due to "silhouette sign" effect. In cases of lung consolidation apart from lung opacity an "air bronchogram" is well seen. There is no lung volume loss in consolidation. Moreover, neither the signs of push nor the signs of pull are seen (Fig. 3.3). In cases of surgical removal of lung (pneumonectomy) there would be evidence of surgery like rib resection. Table 3.3 shows the differentiating features of common causes of unilateral lung opacity in a chest X-ray.

Table 3.2	Signs of 'push' (to opposite side of the lesion) and signs of 'pull' (toward same side of the lesion)

Structure	Push	Pull
Classic, e.g.	Massive pleural effusion	Lobar collapse
Trachea	Displaced to opposite side	Displaced to same side
Mediastinum	Displaced to opposite side	Displaced to same side
Ipsilateral hilum	Displaced to opposite side	Displaced to same side
Intercostal space	Widened	Narrowed
Pulmonary vessels	Not seen	Crowded
Diaphragm	Ipsilateral side depressed	Ipsilateral dome pulled up
Fissure	Not seen	Pulled

Note:
1. Massive pleural effusion shows all signs of "push" to opposite side. For example right sided massive pleural effusion may show signs of "push" to opposite side, i.e. left side.
2. Lobar collapse of lung shows all signs of "pull" towards the same side. For example when there is a right side upper lobe collapse, signs of pull are seen in right side only.

The trachea can be either pulled or pushed, almost always by one of three processes (one that pulls, other that pushes). A right-sided pleural effusion will push the trachea and mediastinum to the opposite side, that is left side. Similarly, a left-sided tension pneumothorax will push the mediastinum to the right, as air builds up in the left pleural space and cannot be released. On the other hand, if there is collapse on the left side, this will pull the trachea and mediastinum to the ipsilateral side, that is, left side. Most other processes (consolidation, non-tension pneumothorax, etc) have little effect on the mediastinum.Therefore, if the mediastinum is shifted in a chest X-ray, then one needs to think of these two lesions (pleural collections and fibrosis) first and look for them.

Massive Pleural Effusion

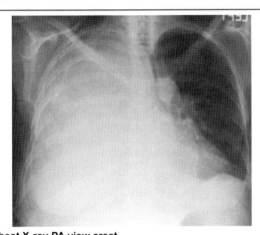 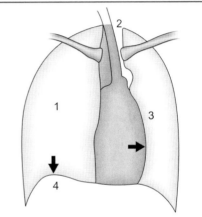

Chest X-ray PA view erect
Opacity right hemithorax
Right diaphragm dome obscured
Right cardiac border obscured
No air bronchogram/bronchovascular markings
Signs of push–mediacstinal shift to left tracheal shift to left widened, i.e. spaces
Increased thoracic volume right side

Signs of push-opposite side
1. Opacity right hemithorax
2. Tracheal shift to left side
3. Mediastinal shift to left-black arrow
4. Right diaphragm dome obscured-black arrow
5. Right cardiac border obscured
Right massive pleural effusion in tension

Fig. 3.1: Chest X-ray showing massive pleural effusion

Massive Lung Collapse

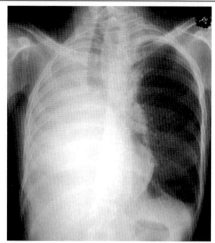

Chest X-ray PA view erect
Homogenous opacity right side thorax
No bronchovascular marking in right
No air bronchogram
Tracheal shift to right
Cardiac (mediastinal) shift to right
Crowding of ribs right
Right diaphragm dome and
Right cardiac border obscured

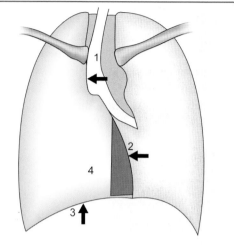

Signs of pull–same side
Right lung collapse
1. Tracheal shift to right side—arrow
2. Cardiac shift to right side—arrow
3. Loss of right dome diaphragm outline—arrow
4. Loss of right heart border outline
Massive total collapse right side

Fig. 3.2: Chest X-ray showing massive lung collapse

Massive Consolidation

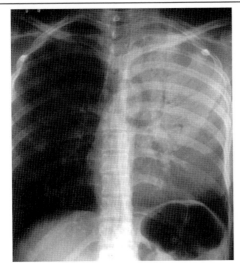 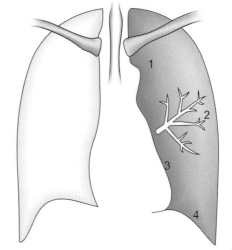

Chest X-ray PA view erect
Homogenous opacity left side thorax
No volume loss
1. Air bronchogram
2. Loss of left heart border silhouette
3. Left dome diaphragm well seen
4. No evidence of push/pull
5. Normal CP angles

No signs of push/pull
1. Homogenous opacity left side thorax
2. Classic airbronchogram
3. Loss of left heart border silhouette
4. Left diaphragm dome well seen
Consolidation left lung upper lobe including lingular segment

Fig. 3.3: Chest X-ray showing massive consolidation

Post-pneumonectomy (Fig. 3.4)

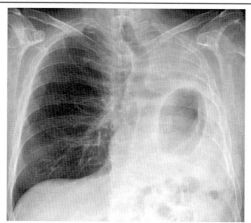 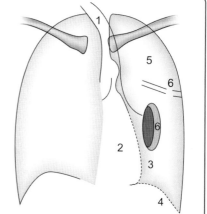

Left side post-pneumonectomy
Evidence of rib resection left side
Opacity left side thorax
Reduced left side thoracic volume
Marked signs of pull
tracheal shift to left
mediastinal shift to left
crowding of left side ribs
left heart border obscured
left diaphragm dome obscured

Signs of pull
1. Tracheal shift to left side
2. Mediastinal shift to left
3. Left heart border obscured
4. Left diaphragm dome obscured
5. Opacity left hemithorax
6. Air trapped postoperative complication
7. Rib resection-evidence of surgery
S/P post-pneumonectomy left lung

Fig. 3.4: Chest X-ray showing post-pneumonectomy changes

Table 3.3	Differential diagnosis of common causes of unilateral lung opacity			
	Parameter	*Pleural effusion*	*Collapse*	*Consolidation*	*Post-pneumonectomy*
1.	Tracheal shift	Opposite side	Same side	No shift	Same side
2.	Mediastinal shift	Opposite side	Same side	No shift	Same side
3.	Thoracic volume	Increased	Reduced	Normal	Reduced
4.	Signs of push	Seen	No	No	No
5.	Signs of pull	No	Seen	No	Seen
6.	Air bronchogram	No	± Minimal	Marked	No
7.	Costophrenic recess	Full, effaced, blunted	Normal	Normal	Normal
8.	Evidence of surgery	Nil	Nil	NIL	Yes, rib resection

Table 3.3 shows the main differentiating features of common conditions that produce unilateral lung opacity.

Unilateral Lung Opacity Involving Part of Lung

There are several common pathologies that cause unilateral lung opacity, involving part of the lung; either a lobe or a brochopulmonary segment. In order to make a quick diagnosis, it is better to categorize them as those producing.

- Well-defined opacity involving lung
- Ill-defined opacities involving lung
- Hilum-based opacities.

Common examples of those producing well-defined opacities involving lung are consolidation, collapse, masses, pleural effusion; those producing ill-defined opacities involving lungs are fibrosis, pleural thickening; those producing hila-based opacities are lymphadenopathy.

Each of these conditions will be discussed based on their X-ray appearances. Each X-ray is accompanied by a corresponding line diagram in order to emphasize clear understanding of the salient X-ray findings. Brief notes on each of these diseases is given.

Well-defined Series

Lobar Consolidation (Fig. 3.5)

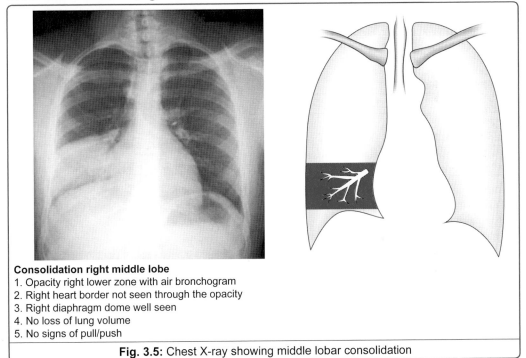

Consolidation right middle lobe
1. Opacity right lower zone with air bronchogram
2. Right heart border not seen through the opacity
3. Right diaphragm dome well seen
4. No loss of lung volume
5. No signs of pull/push

Fig. 3.5: Chest X-ray showing middle lobar consolidation

Pneumonia

Pneumonia is an airspace disease and manifests as lung consolidation. The airspaces are filled with bacteria or other microorganisms and pus. Other causes of airspace filling not distinguishable radiographically would be fluid (inflammatory), cells (bronchoalveolar cancer), protein (alveolar proteinosis) and blood (pulmonary hemorrhage). Pneumonia is not associated with volume loss. Sometimes, the lobe swells up initially (well seen in *Klebsiella pneumonia*) and may shrink slightly later, if there is significant secretions in the airway causing some obstruction. Pneumonia caused by bacteria, viruses, *Mycoplasma* and fungi all appear as

Upper Lobe Consolidation (Fig. 3.6)

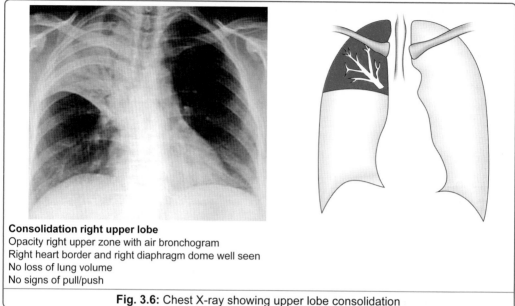

Consolidation right upper lobe
Opacity right upper zone with air bronchogram
Right heart border and right diaphragm dome well seen
No loss of lung volume
No signs of pull/push

Fig. 3.6: Chest X-ray showing upper lobe consolidation

consolidation. The X-ray findings of pneumonia are airspace opacity, involving a lobe (lobar consolidation), or interstitial opacities (bronchopneumonia). There is usually considerable overlap. Pneumonia may have an associated parapneumonic effusion.

Summary of chest X-ray findings in consolidation:
- A density corresponding to a segment or lobe
- An airbronchogram
- No significant loss of lung volume, no signs of push or pull
- Sympathetic pleural effusion (synpneumonic) may be seen.

The types of pneumonia sometimes characteristic on chest X-ray are (Table 3.4):
- Lobar—classically Pneumococcal pneumonia, entire lobe is consolidated and air bronchograms commonly seen.
- Lobular—often *Staphlococcus*, multifocal, patchy, sometimes without air bronchograms.
- Interstitial—Viral or *Mycoplasma*; latter starts perihilar and can become confluent and/or patchy as disease progresses, no air bronchograms.
- Aspiration pneumonia—follows gravitational flow of aspirated contents; impaired consciousness, post anesthesia, common in alcoholics, debilitated, demented patients; usually anerobic (*Bacteroides* and *Fusobacterium*).
- Diffuse pulmonary infections—community acquired (*Mycoplasma*, resolves spontaneoulsy) nosocomial (*Pseudomonas*, debilitated, mechanical ventilation patients, high mortality rate, patchy opacities, cavitation, ill-defined nodular) immunocompromised host (bacterial, fungal, PCP).

Complication of Pneumonic Consolidation Seen in Chest X-ray

1. Cavitation types are:
   a. Lung abscess single, well-defined mass, often with air fluid level

Table 3.4 | Summary of radiographic clues to the etiology of pneumonia

	X-ray finding		Most probable microbe
1.	Round pneumonia	1.	*Streptococcus pneumoniae*
2.	Complete lobar consolidation	2.	*Streptococcus pneumoniae* and *Klebsiella pneumoniae* *Mycobacterium tuberculosis*
3.	Lobar enlargement	3.	*Klebsiella pneumoniae*, *Hemophilus influenza*, *Staphylococcus aureus*, Gram-negative anerobes
4.	Interstitial pneumonia	4.	Viral, *Mycoplasma pneumonia*
5.	Septic emboli, bronchopleural fistula	5.	*Staphylococcus aureus*, Gram-negative anerobes
6.	Empyema	6.	*Mycobacterium tuberculosis*, *Staphylococcus aureus*, Gram-negative anerobes, *Streptococcus*
7.	Cavitation	7.	*Klebsiella pneumoniae*, Gram-negative anerobes
8.	Pulmonary gangrene	8.	*Mycobacterium tuberculosis*, *E. coli*
9.	Pneumatoceles	9.	*Staphylococcus aureus*, *Mycobacterium tuberculosis*, Measles, *Hemophilus influenza*
10.	Lymphadenopathy	10.	*M. tuberculosis*, fungi, virus, *Mycoplasma pneumoniae*

   b. Necrotizing pneumonia, small lucencies or cavities
   c. Pulmonary gangrene, sloughed lung
2. Pneumatoceles
   – Subpleural collections of air that result from alveolar rupture
   – Thin-walled, seen in children; organisms usually *Staphylococcal aureus*
3. Hilar and mediastinal adenopathy
4. Pleural effusion and empyema
5. Other complications
   – ARDS
   – Bronchiectasis
   – Recurrent pneumonitis, unresolved pneumonia.

❏ LOBAR COLLAPSE SERIES

The pathological entities collapse and consolidation produce increased radiographic density. Sometimes it may be difficult to differentiate the two. The Table 3.5 shows some features that distinguish collapse from consolidation. Both collapse and consolidation may coexist in certain situations, especially malignancy.

❏ COLLAPSE/ATELECTASIS

The synonym collapse is often used interchangeably with atelectasis.

   Atelectasis is collapse or incomplete expansion of the lung or part of the lung with loss of lung volume. This is one of the most common findings on a chest X-ray (Fig. 3.7). It is most often caused by an endobronchial lesion, such as mucus plug or tumor or foreign body (active

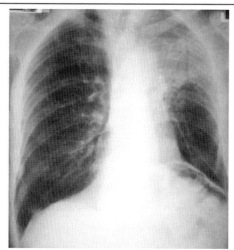

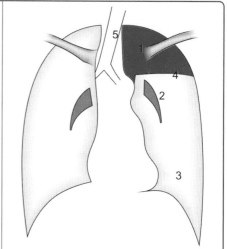

Left upper lobar collapse
Opacity in left upper lobe region
Faint air bronchogram seen in that opacity
Reduction in lung volume signs of pull
Mediastinal shift to left (trachea and heart)
Left hilum abnormally high up
Left diaphragm dome pulled up, lossm of normal doming
Crowding of ribs in left upper zone
Left lower zone vasculature is distorted

1. Opacity left upper zone
2. Left hilum pulled up
3. Left diaphragm dome pulled up (tenting)
4. Crowded ribs
5. Tracheal shift
Signs of local pull, reduction in focal lung volume

Fig. 3.7: Lobar collapse—left upper lobe

Table 3.5 | Differentiating collapse from consolidation

	Finding	Collapse	Consolidation
1.	Shape	Linear, wedge-shaped	Confined to lobe/bronchopulmonary segment
2.	Air bronchogram	May be present	Always present
3.	Lung volume loss	Present	Absent
4.	Signs of pull	Present, same side	Absent
5.	Apex at hilum	Yes	Apex not centered at hilum

collapse). It can also be caused by extrinsic compression centrally by a mass such as lymph nodes or peripheral compression by pleural effusion (passive collapse). An unusual type of atelectasis is cicatricial and is secondary to scarring, TB, or status post radiation.

Atelectasis is reduced inflation of all or part of the lung. The classical primary finding in chest X-ray is reduced volume accompanied by increased opacity in the affected part of the lung. The opacity is often wedge-shaped, with apex pointing toward the hilum. Atelectasis is often associated with abnormal displacement of fissures, bronchi, vessels, diaphragm, hilum, heart, or mediastinum toward the site and side of collapse as secondary indirect signs. These

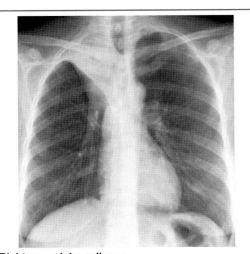

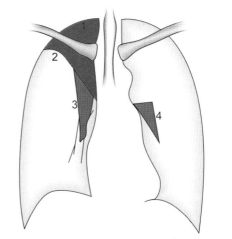

Right upper lobe collapse
There is a triangular opacity in right upper lobe.
The minor fissure and right hilum are markedly pulled up.
Note the crowding of ribs in right upper zone.

1. Collapsed right upper lobe signs of pull due to reduction in lung volume
2. Minor fissure pulled up
3. Right hilum pulled up
4. Normal left hilum

Fig. 3.8: Lobar collapse—right upper lobe

are the classical signs of "pull". Hilar elevation in upper lobe collapse or depression in lower lobe collapse may be seen.

The distribution can be lobar, segmental, or subsegmental. Atelectasis is often qualified by descriptors such as linear, discoid, or plate-like, depending upon the shape.

There may be compensatory hyperinflation of adjacent lobes, segmental and subsegmental collapse may show linear, curvilinear, wedge-shaped opacities.

If a lobe or BPS has collapsed completely, it may be radiographically invisible. An occluding right bronchial lesion results in total collapse of right lung, which has virtually disappeared. Under these circumstances, one has to rely on ancillary radiographic changes to make the diagnosis—signs of pull (Fig. 3.8).

Summary of the Radiographic Signs of Collapse

There are three categories of radiographic signs that contribute to the recognition of lobar collapse:
1. The shadow created by the abnormal lobe itself.
2. Loss of normal lines and shadows. The lines created by anatomical structures will become blurred, if abnormal non-aerated lung collapses against them. For example, the medial part of the respective hemidiaphragm becomes indistinct in the presence of collapse of one or other lower lobe. Similarly, there is loss (or blurring) of the respective heart border in middle lobe or lingula collapse, the paravertebral structures become indistinct in lower lobe collapse and so does the right upper mediastinum in right upper lobe collapse.

3. 'Shift of normal structures'. Signs of pull—the hilar shadows are pulled downward by corresponding lower lobe collapse and upward by shrinking upper lobes.

Signs indicating loss of lung volume (signs of pull toward ipsilateral side) classically seen in collapse are:
a. Tracheal pulled toward same side
b. Mediastinum shifted toward same side
c. Ipsilateral hilar position will change depending upon which lobe is involved
d. Ipsilateral fissure displaced depending upon which lobe is involved
e. Ipsilateral diaphragm pulled up
f. Ipsilateral ribs crowded.

Direct Signs of Collapse

• Displaced septa—a most reliable sign
• Loss of aeration
• Vascular and bronchial signs of crowding.

Indirect Signs of Collapse

• Elevation of a leaf of diaphragm
• Shift of the mediastinal structures toward the side of the affected lobe
• Ipsilateral decrease in size of the thoracic cage
• Compensatory hyperaeration of the uninvolved lobes
• Hilar displacement—most important indirect sign of collapse.

Causes of Collapse

• *Intrinsic mass:* Primary or metastatic neoplasms or eroding lymph nodes
• *Intrinsic stenosis:* TB, inflammatory processes, fracture of a bronchus
• *Extrinsic pressure:* Enlarged lymph nodes, mediastinal tumor, aortic aneurysm
• *Bronchial plugging:* For mucus accumulation.

Types of Collapse

1. Resorption/obstructive/active atelectasis occurs when communication between the trachea and alveoli is obstructed:
   – May be intrinsic, caused by a tumor, foreign body, inflammatory disease, heavy secretions
   – Extrinsic pressure on bronchi caused by tumor or enlarged nodes or bronchial constriction secondary to inflammatory disease
2. Passive atelectasis caused by:
   – Intrapleural abnormalities
   – Caused by space occupying process that can compress the lung
   – Pneumothorax, pleural fluid, diaphragmatic elevation, herniation of the abdominal viscera into the thorax, large intrathoracic tumors

3. Compressive atelectasis:
   - Intrapulmonary abnormalities
   - Is a secondary effect of compression of normal lung by a primary, space-occupying abnormality
   - Bullous emphysema, lobar emphysema
4. Adhesive atelectasis:
   - Occurs when the luminal surfaces of the alveolar walls stick together
   - Hyaline membrane disease, pulmonary embolism, acute radiation pneumonitis, uremia
5. Cicatrization atelectasis:
   - Is primarily the result of fibrosis and scar tissue formation in the interalveolar and interstitial space
   - Classic cause of cicatrizing atelectasis is tuberculosis and histoplasmosis.

Special Forms of Collapse

Golden's "S" Sign

An unusual type of right upper lobe collapse occurs when a hilar mass obstructs the major bronchus (Fig. 3.9). As expected, there is opacity with volume loss in right upper lobe collapse. But the horizontal fissure shows an unusual sigmoid shape with the medial end fixed by the hilar mass and only the lateral end pulled up. The proximal convexity of the horizontal fissure is due to a mass, and the distal concavity is due to atelectasis. The hilar mass fixes the medial part of horizontal fissure and prevents its ascent upward. Only the lateral part of the horizontal fissure is pulled up due to atelectasis. This unusual shape of horizontal fissure is called as Golden's "S" sign and is highly suggestive of malignancy.

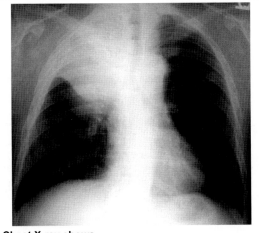

Chest X-ray shows
1. Collapse of right upper lobe
2. S-shaped minor fissure
3. Right hilar mass

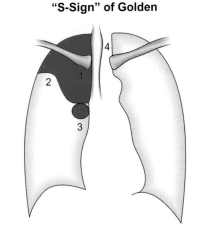

"S-Sign" of Golden

1. Opacity due to collapse right upper lobe
2. S-shaped minor fissure shift
3. Right hilar mass
4. Tracheal shift to right

Fig. 3.9: Chest X-ray to show Golden's "S" sign

Luftsichel Sign

The left lung lacks a middle lobe and therefore a minor fissure, so left upper lobe atelectasis presents a different picture from that of the right upper lobe collapse. The result is predominantly anterior shift of the upper lobe in left upper lobe collapse, with loss of the left upper cardiac border. The expanded lower lobe will migrate to a location both superior and posterior to the upper lobe in order to occupy the vacated space. As the lower lobe expands, it produces lucency outlining the aortic knob unusually clear. This is called as "Luftsichel sign".

In the X-ray (Figs 3.10 and 3.11) with left upper lobe collapse, the superior segment of the left lower lobe, which is positioned between the aortic arch and the collapsed left upper lobe, is hyperinflated. This aerated segment of left lower lobe is hyperlucent and shaped like a sickle, where it outlines the aortic arch on the frontal chest radiograph. This periaortic lucency has been termed the luftsichel sign, derived from the German words luft (air) and sichel (sickle).

Increased tranlucency in left lung mid and lower zone. There is wedge shaped ground glass haziness in left upper zone with pulled up left hilum. Lucenct band like area is seen in left upper zone between above mentioned wedge-shaped ground glass haziness and arch of aorta. Wedge-shaped ground glass haziness in left upper zone represents left upper lobe collapse. Lucenct band like area in left upper zone—represents hyperinflatted superior segment of left lower lobe. This is known as 'Luftsichel'.

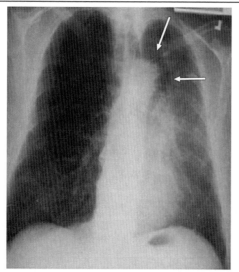 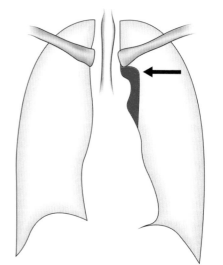

Note the mediastinal shift to left. The white arrows point toward the unusual lucency around the aortic knob. Note the elevated left dome of diaphragm. Overinflated right lung (compensatory emphysema).	The black arrow point toward the unusual lucency around the aortic knob.

Fig. 3.10: Chest X-ray showing Luftsichel sign

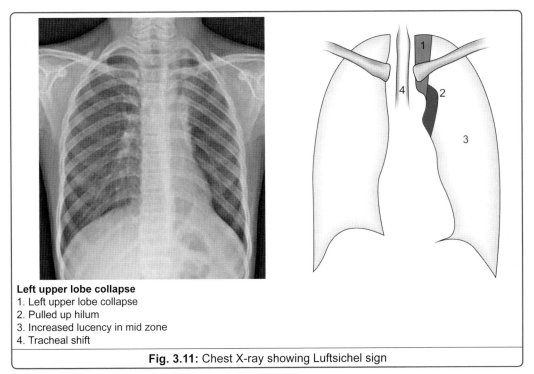

Left upper lobe collapse
1. Left upper lobe collapse
2. Pulled up hilum
3. Increased lucency in mid zone
4. Tracheal shift

Fig. 3.11: Chest X-ray showing Luftsichel sign

❑ COLLAPSE OF INDIVIDUAL LOBES (TABLE 3.6)

Right Upper Lobe

Right upper lobe atelectasis is easily detected as the lobe migrates superomedially toward the apex and mediastinum. The minor fissure elevates and the inferior border of the collapsed lobe is a well demarcated curvilinear border arcing from the hilum towards the apex with inferior concavity. Due to reactive hyperaeration of the lower lobe, the lower lobe artery will often be displaced superiorly on a frontal view.

Right Middle Lobe

Right middle lobe atelectasis may cause minimal changes on the frontal chest film. A loss of definition of the right heart border is the key finding. The horizontal and lower portion of the major fissures start to approximate with increasing opacity leading to a wedge of opacity pointing to the hilum.

Right Lower Lobe

Silhouetting of the right hemidiaphragm and a triangular density posteromedially are common signs of right lower lobe atelectasis. Right lower lobe atelectasis can be distinguished from right middle lobe atelectasis by the persistence of the right heart border.

Table 3.6 | Radiographic features in various lung lobe collapse

Part	Right side	Left side
Entire	Homogenous density right hemithorax Mediastinal shift to right Right hemithorax smaller Right heart and diaphragmatic silhouette are not identifiable	Homogenous density left hemithorax Mediastinal shift to left Left hemithorax smaller Diaphragm and heart silhouette are not identifiable
Upper lobe	Density in the right upper lung field Transverse fissure pulled up Right hilum pulled up Smaller right hemithorax	Mediastinal shift to left Density left upper lung field Loss of aortic knob and left hilar silhouettes Left hilum pulled up
Middle lobe	Vague density in right lower lung field (almost a normal film) Movement of transverse fissure down Right heart silhouette are not identifiablett	
Lower lobe	Density in right lower lung field Indistinct right diaphragm Right heart silhouette retained Transverse fissure moved down Right hilum moved down	Inhomogeneous cardiac density Triangular retrocardiac density Left hilum pulled down Indistinct left diaphragm

Pleural Effusion

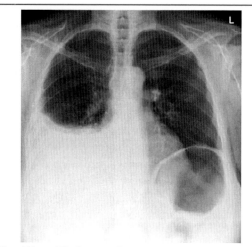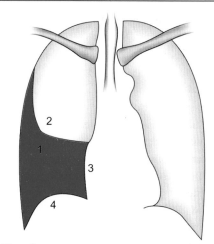

Chest X-ray PA view erect	Line diagram
Opacity right lower zone Opacity centered at right CP angle the opacity has concave upper border Opacity extends along right costal pleura Right diaphragm dome obscured Right cardiac border obscured No air bronchogram No signs of pull/push	1. Opacity right lower zone 2. The opacity has concave upper border 3. Right cardiac border obscured 4. Right diaphragm dome obscured Moderate right pleural effusion

Fig. 3.12: Chest X-ray showing right pleural effusion

Pleural Effusion

This is accumulation of fluid in the potential pleural space between visceral and parietal layers. All types of fluid—blood, pus, chyle, transudate, exudate-appear white in radiography.

There needs to be at least 75 mL of pleural fluid in order to blunt the costophrenic angle on the lateral chest radiograph, and 200 mL on the posteroanterior chest radiograph. Pleural effusions typically have a meniscus visible on an erect chest radiograph, but loculated effusions (as occur with an empyema) may have a lenticular shape (the fluid making an obtuse angle with the chest wall).

The classical signs of moderate are homogeneous opacification of the lower chest with obliteration of the costophrenic angle and the hemidiaphragm. The superior margin of the opacity is concave to the lung and is higher laterally than medially. Above and medial to the meniscus, there is a hazy increase in opacity owing to the presence of fluid posterior and anterior to the lungs.

On supine chest radiographs, which are commonly used in the intensive care setting, moderate to large pleural effusions may appear as a homogenous increase in density spread over the lower lung fields. Apparent elevation of the hemidiaphragm, lateral displacement of the dome of the diaphragm, or increased distance between the apparent left hemidiaphragm and the gastric air bubble suggests subpulmonic effusions. Additional signs include haziness of the diaphragmatic margin, blunting of the costophrenic angle, a pleural cap to the lung apex, thickening of the minor fissure and widening of the paraspinal interface.

Pleural thickening may also cause blunting of the costophrenic angle, but is distinguished from pleural fluid by the fact that it occurs as a linear shadow ascending vertically and clinging to the ribs, without showing any fluid shift.

Bilateral pleural effusions tend to be transudates because they develop secondary to generalized changes that affect both pleural cavities equally. Some bilateral effusions are exudates, however, and this is seen with metastatic disease, lymphoma, pulmonary embolism, rheumatoid disease, systemic lupus erythematosus (SLE), post-cardiac injury syndrome, myxoedema and some ascites-related effusions.

Massive effusions cause dense opacification of the hemithorax with contralateral mediastinal shift. Absence of mediastinal shift with a large effusion raises the strong possibility of obstructive collapse of the ipsilateral lung or extensive pleural malignancy, such as may be seen with mesothelioma or metastatic carcinoma (lung or breast), and may also occur in heart failure, cirrhosis, tuberculosis, empyema and trauma.

Right-sided effusions are typically associated with ascites, heart failure and liver abscess, and left effusions with pancreatitis, pericarditis, esophageal rupture and aortic dissection.

Pleural effusion is common in heart failure and tends to be more frequent and larger on the right. All types of pericardial disease may be associated with pleural effusion which is predominantly left-sided. Pulmonary embolism is commonly associated with pleural effusion which is seen in 25–50% of cases.

Both acute and chronic pancreatitis are associated with pleural effusions which have high amylase levels. In acute pancreatitis, exudative and often blood-stained effusions form in 15% of patients, particularly on the left side where the diaphragm is closely related to the pancreatic tail. Associated elevation of the hemidiaphragm and basal lung consolidation are common. In chronic pancreatitis, effusions tend to be large and recurrent and patients present with dyspnoea, unlike effusions in acute pancreatitis in which abdominal symptoms predominate. The pathogenesis of pleural effusion in chronic pancreatitis is fistula formation following ductal rupture.

Pleural effusion is common with subphrenic abscess and amoebic liver abscess. The effusion is often accompanied by basal lung collapse and consolidation, an elevated hemidiaphragm and a subdiaphragmatic air-fluid level. Pleural effusion may occur in a number of renal conditions. Exudative effusions may be seen in uremia and are often accompanied by pericarditis. Empyema is a suppurative exudate usually parapneumonic. Less commonly it is caused by transdiaphragmatic extension of a liver abscess or by bronchopleural fistula.

Hemothorax

On the plain chest radiograph an acute hemothorax is indistinguishable from other pleural fluid collections. Once the blood clots, there is a tendency for loculation and occasionally a fibrin body will form. Pleural thickening and calcification are recognized sequelae. The most common cause of hemothorax is trauma, but it is seen in a number of other conditions, including ruptured aortic aneurysm, pneumothorax, extramedullary hemopoiesis and coagulopathies.

Lung Mass Single Large

Lung Masses

The most common cause of lung mass in an elderly person is malignancy. A lung mass is one which is large and well-defined and does not confine to a lobe and measures 3 cm size. In a chest X-ray, it may appear as a solitary peripheral mass (Fig. 3.13). Central location is seen in 40% of cases. The mass can be smooth or irregular in outline and can cavitate. Satellite nodules may be present. There may be hilar, paratracheal and/or mediastinal lymphadenopathy. Direct spread may result in rib destruction and extrathoracic extension. There may be distant rib metastases.

Other CXR presentations include patchy consolidation that fails to respond to antibiotics (commonly BAC), pleural effusions, bronchoceles and lung collapse, which may be partial or complete (lobar/segmental).

Pancoast Tumor (Fig. 3.14)

This is also known as superior sulcus carcinoma. It is a squamous-cell carcinoma. Most common type of lung CA to cause hypercalcemia.

Radiologic Features

Two-thirds in central:
Atelectasis of lung or lobe Postobstructive pneumonitis

- One-third peripheral thick-walled, cavitary mass solidary nodule
- Other CXR findings—unilateral apical pleural thickening/mass. The mass lesion may cavitate. Hilar enlargement secondary to lymphadenopathy. May be rib destruction and extrathoracic soft tissue mass lesion.

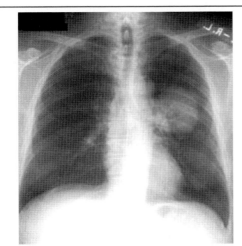 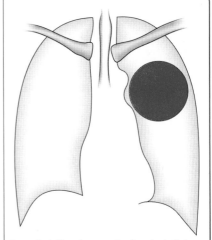

A well defined oval shaped mass lesion in left parahilar region, mass has well-defined borders. Since the hilum is seen through the mass, the mass is not in plane with the hilum (Hilum overlay sign). The mass is abutting the left main bronchus. Since the posterior ribs do not show any erosion, the mass in this patient is anteriorly placed

A well-defined mass lesion in left lung midzone-Blue mass

Fig. 3.13: Chest X-ray showing a mass lesion

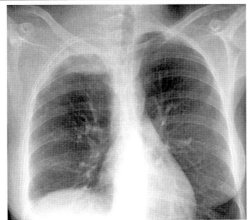

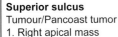
Superior sulcus
Tumour/Pancoast tumor
1. Right apical mass
2. Soft tissue extension
3. Paralysed right dome

Fig. 3.14: Chest X-ray lung mass showing pancoast tumor

Clinical Features

Pain, Horner's syndrome, bone destruction atrophy of hand muscles, invasion chest wall, base of neck, brachial plexus, vertebral bodies and spinal canal, sympathetic ganglion, subclavian artery.

Peripheral Lung Carcinoma (Fig. 3.15)

1. The cell type large-cell undifferentiated carcinoma
   Large bulky peripheral mass, necrosis, pleural involvement with effusion, more aggressive and spread early > 4 cm.
   Paraneoplastic syndromes associated with bronchogenic carcinoma, hypercalcemia, ectopic adrenocorticotropic hormone production, syndrome of inappropriate secretion of antidiuretic hormone, Eaton-Lambert syndrome (peripheral neuropathy with myasthenia-like symptoms), acanthosis nigricans, hypertrophic osteoarthropathy
2. Adenocarcinoma
   Peripheral with lobulated or irregular margins, solitary nodule or mass, spiculated border, pleural retraction or tethering, hilar or perihilar mass, Parenchymal mass with hilar or mediastinal lymphadenopathy

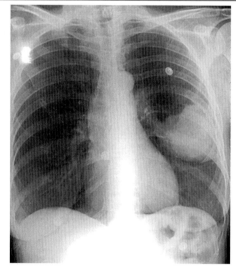

Peripheral placed lung mass
The mass is well defined
In left mid zone, abutting the pleural surface. There is a continuity
with left hilum, which is enlarged.

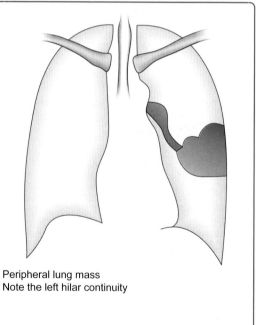

Peripheral lung mass
Note the left hilar continuity

Fig. 3.15: Chest X-ray lung mass showing peripheral lung carcinoma

3. Bronchioloalveolar carcinoma (alveolar cell carcinoma)

Solitary nodule most common, hazy, ill-defined, air bronchogram consolidation or multiple nodules

4. Small cell carcinoma—Most common lung CA to cause superior vena cava obstruction, Cushing's syndrome and secretion of inappropriate antidiuretic hormone (SIADH).

Arises in association with proximal airways, lobar and main bronchi, centrally located tumor hilar or perihilar mass massive adenopathy, often bilateral, Rare-peripheral nodule.

Lung Mass—Multiple and Large

Lung Secondaries

This is the most common cause of multiple masses in lung. The masses are well defined with varying sizes. In known case of malignancy elsewhere in the body, any lung mass is a secondary unless otherwise proved.

Metastatic disease—hematogenous spread

Both lungs, lower lobes, periphery, round, well marginated, variable doubling times, Ca^{++} in primary bone and cartilage tumors, mucinous adenocarcimonas, cavitation in metastatic squamous cell CA, solitary pulmonary nodule, renal cell carcinoma.

Metastatic disease—lymphangitic spread

Primary sites—lung, breast, upper-abdominal malignancy, more commonly bilateral, radiographic features, reticulonadar pattern, Kerley B lines, pleural effusion (60%), adenopathy (25%) (Fig. 3.16).

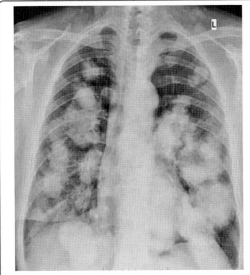

Typical cannon balls
Multiple, well defined round masses seen in both lung zones. The masses are of different sizes

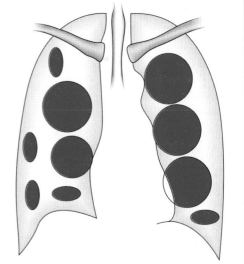

In a patient with known malignancy elsewhere in the body these finding are secondaries unless otherwise proved

Fig. 3.16: Chest X-ray showing multiple large masses

Metastatic disease – endobronchial metastases
Site of primary malignancy: Kidney, melanoma, thyrpoid, breast, colon; radiographic features: atelectasis, hilar mass.

Metastatic disease – intrathoracic adenopathy
Sites of primary malignancy: genitourinary, head and neck, breast, skin (melanoma); radiographic features: adenopathy ± parenchymal metastases.

Metastases other characteristics
- Metastatic disease within the chest represents spread to the lung, pleura, bones and soft tissues.
- Lung metastases are common, occurring in 30% of all malignancies.
- Common cancers include breast, kidney, colorectal and prostate.
- Lung metastases are prominent in rarer malignancies such as osteosarcoma, thyroid cancer and melanoma.
- It can present as a solitary lung nodule (60% chance of malignant lesion), multiple lung nodules, diffuse air space opacification or diffuse reticulonodular change (lymphangitis carcinomatosis).

Different radiological features
Solitary or multiple rounded lung lesions.
- They may be calcified (osteosarcoma, breast, thyroid and mucinous adenocarcinoma).
- They may be small (thyroid, breast, prostate, choriocarcinoma).
- Cavitating (squamous cell, colon, melanoma, transitional cell carcinoma).
- Hemorrhagic (choriocarcinoma, melanoma, thyroid).
- Endobronchial (lung, lymphoma, breast, renal or colorectal carcinoma).
- Air space opacification (adenocarcinoma of the breast, ovary or GI tract).
- Lymphadenopathy may be present.
- Septal lines, irregular fissural nodularity—lymphangitis (breast, colon, pancreas and stomach).

Lung Carcinoma

The six cell types of primary lung carcinoma are as follows:
- Adenocarcinoma—(35-50%) Peripheral masses
- Squamous cell carcinoma—(30%) Central, with hilar involvement, cavitation is common, slow growing
- Small cell—(15-20%) Central, cavitation is rare, hilar and mediastinal masses often the dominant feature, rapid growth and early metastases
- Large cell—(10-15%) Peripheral masses large, cavitation present
- Bronchaveolar—(3%) Peripheral, rounded appearance, pneumonia-like infiltrate (air bronchograms)
- Carcinoid—(less than 1%) Typically a well defined endobronchial lesion or present as a solitary.

Lung cancers are unresectable once they have progressed to a TNM staging of any of the below.
- T4—Invasion of the mediastinum or involvement of the heart, great vessels, trachea, esophagus, vertebral body, or carina; or neoplasia associated with a malignant pleural or pericardial effusion, or satellite nodules in the same lobe

- N3—Metastasis to contralateral mediastinal and hilar nodes, ipsilateral or contralateral scalene or supraclavicular nodes
- M1—distant metastasis present

Lung Nodule—Single Small

Any pulmonary lesion represented in a radiograph by a sharply defined, discrete, nearly circular opacity 2–30 mm in diameter is called a nodule.

A solitary nodule in the lung can be totally innocuous or potentially a fatal lung cancer. A nodule that is unchanged for two years is almost certainly benign. If the nodule is completely calcified or has central or stippled calcium it is benign. Nodules with irregular calcifications or those that are off center should be considered suspicious, and need to be worked up further.

Some 40% of SPN are malignant, with other common lesions being granulomas and benign tumours. A nodule is assessed for its size, shape and outline and for the presence of calcification or cavitation. Popcorn type of calcification is typically seen in hamartomas. Granulomas are the most common cause of SPN. Granulomas are well defined, lobulated, frequently calcify, may be multiple, but small in size. Metastasis show varying sizes. AVM may have a feeding vessel and a draining vein.

Benign lung tumors: Hamartomas; 5–8% of SPN

Radiologic features: Solitary well-defined pulmonary nodules, calcification ++ 10 to 15% (Fig. 3.17).

Tuberculoma

This is the most common bacterial infection that can produce a SPN. The X-ray features are round or oval, sharply circumscribed nodule. They are often small, widespread and punctate.

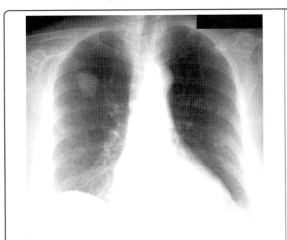 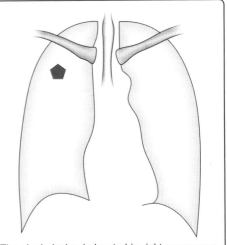

| There is a well defined single lesion, located in the right upper zone. Since the mass lesion did not change its morphology-site, size, shape, etc. compared to the previous X-rays the lesion is more likely to be a benign one. | The single lesion is located in right upper zone. The tumour doubling time was more than two years, hence it is likely to be benign. |

Fig. 3.17: Chest X-ray showing solitary pulmonary nodule (SPN)

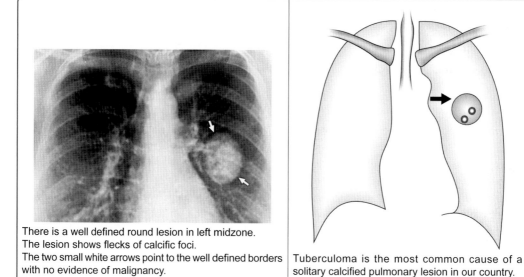

There is a well defined round lesion in left midzone.
The lesion shows flecks of calcific foci.
The two small white arrows point to the well defined borders with no evidence of malignancy. | Tuberculoma is the most common cause of a solitary calcified pulmonary lesion in our country.

Fig. 3.18: Chest X-ray showing tuberculoma in lung

Solitary granulomata, particularly post TB infection, can be large up to several centimetres in diameter. They represent a chronic healed immune reaction, within the lung, to the initial stimulus. Post-infective causes – TB, post varicella pneumonia. Non-infectious causes – inhalation of organic and inorganic chemicals. Central calcification and calcification of hilar lymph nodes may be seen.

Tuberculoma typically appears as a fairly discrete nodule or mass in which repeated extensions of infection have created a core of caseous necrosis surrounded by a mantle of epithelioid cells and collagen with peripheral round cell infiltration. The majority of tuberculomas are less than 3 cm in diameter. Small, discrete shadows in the vicinity of the main lesion (satellite lesions) may be identified in as many as 80% of cases. The tuberculomas are usually smooth in outline but may have a rough edge on CT scans. Calcification is found in 20–30% of the lesions and is usually nodular or diffuse. The presence of benign-looking calcification within the nodule, adjacent tree-in-bud lesions, or satellite nodules may help in differentiating tuberculomas from malignant nodules.

Lung Nodule—Multiple Tiny

Miliary Mottling

Miliary tuberculosis (also known as disseminated tuberculosis) is a form of tuberculosis that is characterized by a wide dissemination into the human body and by the tiny size of the lesions (1–3 mm). Its name comes from a distinctive pattern seen on a chest X-ray of many tiny spots

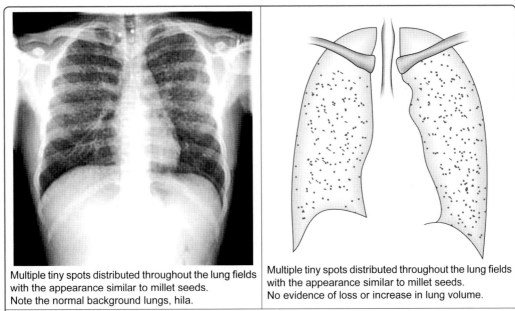

Multiple tiny spots distributed throughout the lung fields with the appearance similar to millet seeds. Note the normal background lungs, hila.

Multiple tiny spots distributed throughout the lung fields with the appearance similar to millet seeds. No evidence of loss or increase in lung volume.

Fig. 3.19: Chest X-ray showing multiple tiny nodules

distributed throughout the lung fields with the appearance similar to millet seeds—thus the term "miliary" tuberculosis.

Miliary tuberculosis may occur as primary TB or may develop years after the initial infection. The disseminated nodules consist of central caseating necrosis and peripheral epithelioid and fibrous tissue. Radiographically, they are not calcified. Chest X-ray findings are typical in 50% of cases. A bright spotlight helps to reveal miliary nodules.

The classic description of millary TB on chest radiographs is of uniform 2 to 3 mm discrete nodules evenly distributed throughout the lung parenchyma (Fig. 3.19). Sometimes, a slight basal predominance may be detected. The presence of lymph-node enlargement is commonly associated with miliary pulmonary TB in children (95% incidence) but less so in adults (12%). Similarly, other evidence of primary TB, including focal parenchymal consolidation, pleural effusion that may represent the source of dissemination, has been shown to be a more frequent finding in children (42%) than in adults (12%).

Pneumoconiosis Characteristics

These represent a spectrum of lung conditions caused by inhalation of inorganic dust particles. The particles overwhelm the lung's defence mechanism and induce a chronic granulomatous reaction. The exposure to the particles occurs over many years.
The resulting lung changes are progressive and irreversible.

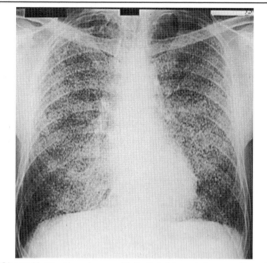
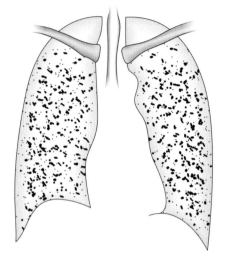

| Chest X-ray showing multiple bright nodules scattered throughout the lung zones. Almost uniformly. The lesions are too bright and too large for them to be called miliary tuberculosis. This is a case of stannosis. | Line diagram showing multiple very dense nodular shadows scattered diffusely, that is, involving all the five lobes of lung. Further the nodules do not show the same size. |

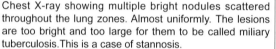

Fig. 3.20: Chest X-ray showing multiple tiny nodules—a case of pneumoconiosis

There are two main subtypes of pneumoconiosis:

Minimal symptoms as the particles are not fibrogenic, e.g. stannosis (tin), baritosis (barium) and siderosis (iron).

Symptomatic due to fibrogenic particles, e.g. silicosis (silica), asbestosis (asbestos) and coal workers' pneumoconiosis.

All the conditions have very similar characteristic clinical and radiological features.

Clinical Features

- May be asymptomatic.
- Nonproductive cough.
- Dyspnea—this is progressive.
- Weight loss, malaise.
- Hypoxia.
- Restrictive lung function.

Radiological Features

CXR: Multiple bilateral 3 to 10 mm nodules present in the upper and mid zones. Some of the nodules coalesce. Different particles produce different density nodules, e.g. stannosis can be very dense. There may be hilar lymphadenopathy some of which show egg shell calcification. There may be fibrotic change and parenchymal distortion.

HRCT: It Demonstrates small nodular opacities, interlobular septal thickening, fibrous parenchymal bands and a ground glass pattern.

Note on asbestosis: The first manifestation of exposure to asbestos is the pleural effusion, occurring within 10 years of exposure. Most are asymptomatic with exudative often bloody effusions. Most spontaneously resolve within a few months though some may persist for years. The pleural plaques tend to develop along the postero- and antero-lateral chest wall and the central tendon of the diaphragm. Plaques are often holly leafed shaped along the chest wall. Asbestosis is dose related and seen in those with continued prolonged exposure to asbestos fibers. Typical radiographic findings are basilar peripheral irregular shaped reticular opacities due to fibrosis and multiple nodules. Asbestos is an independent risk factor for the development of lung carcinoma, especially mesothelioma, equivalent to that of a smoker. If the exposed individual also smokes the risk is multiplicative.

Unilateral "ILL Defined" Lung Opacity Involving Part of Lung

ILL Defined Fibrosis in TB

Tuberculosis

Primary tuberculosis (TB) is the initial infection with *Mycobacterium tuberculosis*.

Post-primary TB is reactivation of a primary focus, or continuation of the initial infection.

Radiographically, TB is represented by consolidation, adenopathy, and pleural effusion. A Ghon focus is an area of consolidation that most commonly occurs in the mid and lower lung zones. A Ghon complex is the addition of hilar adenopathy and thickened minor fissure to a Ghon focus. The classic Ghon complex ocurs only in children.

Radiographic features of post-primary TB include any or all of the following: focal patchy airspace disease "cottonwool" shadows, cavitation, fibrosis, nodal calcification, and flecks of

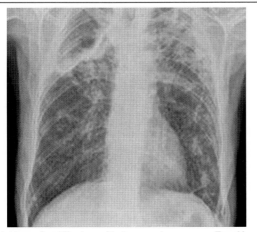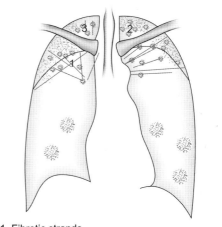

Total loss of architecture of both upper lung zones. Focal loss of lung volume with evidence of local pull signs like pulled up hila, crowding of upper ribs, etc.	1. Fibrotic strands 2. Ill defined infiltrates 3. Predominantly upper lobe involvement.

Fig. 3.21: Chest X-ray showing fibrous-cavernous tuberculosis

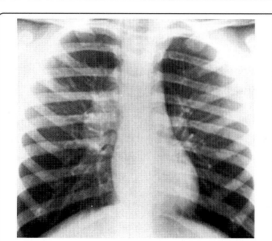

A Ghon focus is an area of consolidation that most commonly occurs in the mid and lower lung zones. A Ghon complex is the addition of hilar adenopathy to and thickened minor fissure to a Ghon focus. The classic Ghon complex occurs only in children.

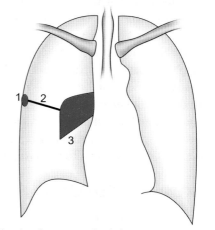

Classic primary complex in lung
1. Sub pleural Ghon tuberculous focus
2. Regional lymphangitis along minor fissure
3. Regional hilar lymphadenopathy

Fig. 3.22: Chest X-ray to show Ghons complex (primary complex) in childhood TB

caseous material, plueral effusion or thickening. The lung parenchymal lesions occur most commonly in the posterior segments of the upper lobes, and superior segments of the lower lobes for reasons not well known.

Fibrosis and cavitation are the hallmarks of adult TB. Fibrosis is not seen in children. Hilar lymphadenopathy is the hallmark of childhood TB. Adult TB can have mediastinal lymphadenopathy, especially when the patient is immunecompromised. Atypical tuberculosis features like involvement of lower/middle lobe, hilar adenopathy, frank consolidation in adults, occur mostly in immunocompromised persons and involve anterior segment of the upper lobes.

With Pleural involvement—effusion and empyema may occur some with bronchopleural fistula. Tuberculoma especially in upper lobe, right side more often than the left is seen.

Primary Complex—Childhood TB

Primary tuberculosis (TB) is the initial infection with *Mycobacterium tuberculosis*.

Post-primary TB is reactivation of a primary focus, or continuation of the initial infection.

Radiographically, TB is represented by consolidation, adenopathy, and pleural effusion. But Ghon's complex is the most common form seen exclusively in children. A Ghon focus is an area of consolidation that most commonly occurs in the mid and lower lung zones. A Ghon complex is the addition of hilar adenopathyto and thickened minor fissure to a Ghon focus. The classic ghon-complex ocurs only in children (Fig. 3.22).

Enlarged hilar and paratracheal nodes most often calcify. Bilateral involvement is seen in approximately 20% of cases. The lymphadenopathy is always associated with ipsilateral parenchymal disease.

Ghon focus, initial focus of parenchymal disease, Ranke complex, combination of Ghon focus and affected lymph nodes. Radiologic manifestations are:

1. Parenchymal involvement air-space consolidation.
   Right upper lobe—most common (adult), right middle lobe—least common
2. Lymph node involvement—hilar and mediastinal—right paratracheal region (children)
3. Airway involvement lobar and right sided atelectasis or consolidation

The differential diagnosis of a disseminated miliary pattern on chest radiograph is extensive. The more common of these include other infections such as the disseminated mycoses, viral pneumonias, inhalational diseases such as silicosis and extrinsic allergic alveolitis, metastatic disease (particularly thyroid carcinoma), and bronchioloalveolar carcinoma.

❑ HILUM BASED OPACITY

Causes of Enlarged HILA

1. Unilateral hilar adenopathy
   a. Neoplasm
   b. Primary tuberculosis
   c. Sarcoidosis (8%)
   d. Primary pulmonary fungal infection
2. Bilateral hilar adenopathy
   a. Sarcoidosis
   b. Lymphoma
   c. False positive
   d. Expiration film
   e. Pulmonary hypertension

Hilar enlargement could be due to an abnormality in any of the three structures which lie at the hilum.

- The pulmonary artery—for example, pulmonary artery hypertension, secondary to mitral valve disease, valvar pulmonary stenosis chronic pulmonary emboli, or primary pulmonary hypertension
- The main bronchus—carcinoma arising in the proximal bronchus
- Enlarged lymph nodes—caused by infection, such as tuberculosis—spread from a primary lung tumor, lymphoma, or sarcoidosis. This is the most common cause of hilar enlargment.

Hilar Lymphadenopathy

Enlargement of the lymph nodes within the lung hilum can be an important finding for underlying pathology.

A differential of possible etiologies can be broken up into three different categories:

- Inflammation (sarcoidosis, silicosis)
- Neoplasm (lymphoma, metastases, bronchogenic carcinoma)
- Infection (tuberculosis, histoplasmosis, infectious mononucleosis).

An important consideration to keep in mind is that since the pulmonary arteries also course through the same area, enlargement of these vessels may be confused with hilar adenopathy.

Table 3.7 | Mediastinal vs pulmonary mass

Mediastinal mass	Pulmonary mass
Epicenter in the mediastinum	Epicenter in lung
Obtuse angle with the lung	Acute angle with the lung
(-) air bronchogram	(+) air bronchogram
Smooth and sharp margins	Irregular margins
Movement with swallowing	Movement with respiration
Bilateral	Unilateral

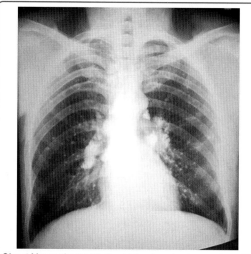 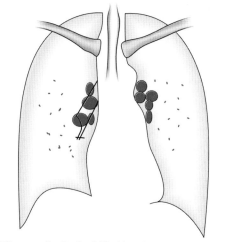

Chest X-ray shows bilateral hilar lymphadenopathy with calcification. There is an evidence of small calcific foci in the lung zones also	Diffuse mediastinal calcified lymphadenopathy, in our country, is always due to tuberculosis

Fig. 3.23: Chest X-ray showing tuberculous lymphadenopathy

Typically, lymphadenopathy has a more lumpy-bumpy appearance, while an enlarged pulmonary artery appears smooth.

Tuberculous Lymphadenopathy

Enlarged hilar and paratracheal nodes most often calcify. Bilateral involvement is seen in approximately 20% of cases. The lymphadenopathy is always associated with ipsilateral parenchymal disease. The lymphadenopathy is asymmetrical, involving any group in mediastinum.

The lymph node in lung parenchyma/interstitium may also be involved, may show calcification. Calcification in tuberculous lymphadenopathy does not rule out active disease.

Sarcoidosis

Bilaterally symmetric enlargement of hilar and paratracheal nodes develops in up to 90% of patients. The outer borders of the enlarged hila are usually lobulated.

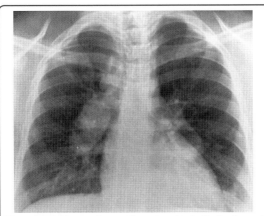 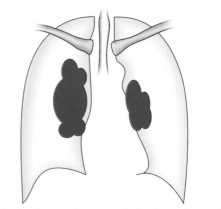

The chest X-ray shows the classic 1, 2, 3 sign of sarcoidosis
1-Right hilar lymphadenopathy
2-Left hilar lymphadenopathy
3-Right paratracheal lymphadenopathy

Note the lumpy, knobby bilateral mediastinal lymphadenopathy.
Pleura is not involved in sarcoidosis, differentiating other causes of lymphadenopathy.

Fig. 3.24: Chest X-ray showing 1,2,3 sign of sarcoidosis

Approximately half the patients have diffuse parenchymal disease. Nodal enlargement often resolves as the parenchymal disease develops, unlike lymphoma or tuberculosis. The bilateral symmetry is unlike tuberculosis, whereas the lack of retrosternal involvement is unlike lymphoma.

enlargement of the right hilar, left hilar, and right paratracheal lymph nodes, producing the classic 1,2,3 pattern of adenopathy. Sometimes chest X-ray may be normal. The staging of sarcoidosis are:

Stage 1–Bilateral hilar and mediastinal lymphadenopathy (particularly right paratracheal and aortopulmonary window nodes).

Stage 2–Lymphadenopathy and parenchymal disease.

Stage 3–Diffuse parenchyma disease only.

Stage 4–Pulmonary fibrosis.

The parenchymal disease involves reticulonodular shadowing in a perihilar, mid zone distribution. There is bronchovascular and fissural nodularity. Rarely air space consolidation or parenchymal bands may also be present. Fibrosis affects the upper zones where the hilar are pulled superiorly and posteriorly. Lymph nodes can demonstrate egg shell calcification.

Lymphoma

Primarily Hodgkin's disease, which often produces asymmetric bilateral hilar adenopathy. There may be pulmonary involvement or pleural effusion. The nodes may calcify after mediastinal irradiation.

Enlargement of all hilar and mediastinal nodes (the anterior mediastinal and retrosternal nodes are frequently affected). Typically bilateral but asymmetric (unilateral node enlargement is very rare).

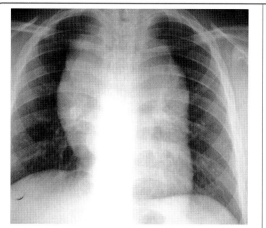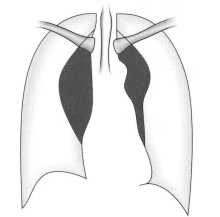

| Chest X-ray showing bilateral massive hilar enlargement. Note the knobby outline, normal cardiac size. Normal lung zones. | Bilateral massive mediastinal lymphadenopathy in a young person is due to lymphoma, unless otherwise proved. |

Fig. 3.25: Chest X-ray showing massive lymphadenopathy of lymphoma

Most common radiographic finding in Hodgkin's disease (visible on the initial chest films of approximately 50% of patients). Pulmonary involvement or pleural effusion occurs in about 30%. Calcification may develop in intrathoracic lymph nodes after mediastinal irradiation.

Hodgkin's Disease

Clinical features
Bimodal age-distribution, young adults, elderlymen, mass in neck or groin

Radiographic features
- 85% thoracic involvement
- Multiple lymph node groups
- Anterior mediastinum most common
- Lung involvement; Primary-lung Hodgkin's rare, nodules, masses
- Perihilar cavitation, air bronchograms
- Egg shell calcification in nodes after radiotherapy.

❑ BILATERAL LUNG OPACITY

Congestive Cardiac Failure (CCF)

Congestive heart failure is one of the most common abnormalities evaluated by CXR. CHF occurs when the heart fails to maintain adequate forward flow. It usually refers to failure of both side of heart-right and left. CHF may progress to pulmonary venous hypertension and pulmonary edema with leakage of fluid into the interstitium, alveoli and pleural space.

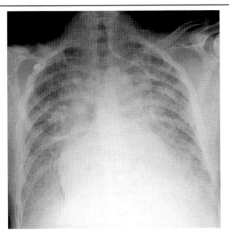

Chest X-ray showing:	The cardiac silhouette is enlarged.
Generalised cardiac enlargement increased CTR	There is bilateral lung opacity radiating from hila
Note the indistinct heart borders, bilateral hilar	region.
enlargement.	The cardiophrenic angles are blunted.
Bilateral perihilar opacities.	

Fig. 3.26: Chest X-ray showing bilateral lung opacities in CCF

The earliest CXR finding of CHF is cardiomegaly, detected as an increased cardiothoracic ratio (>50%). In the pulmonary vasculature of the normal chest, the lower zone pulmonary veins are larger than the upper zone veins due to gravity. In a patient with CHF, the pulmonary capillary wedge pressure rises to the 12-18 mm Hg range and the upper zone veins dilate and are equal in size or larger, this is termed cephalization. With increasing PCWP, (18-24 mm Hg), interstitial edema occurs with the appearance of Kerley B lines. Increased PCWP above this level is alveolar edema, often in a classic perihilar batwing pattern of density. Pleural effusions also often occur. CXR is important in evaluating patients with CHF for development of pulmonary edema and evaluating response to therapy as well.

Once CCF sets in, it is very difficult to determine the precise cause of the failure.

Congestive Cardiac Failure—Kerley B Lines

These are horizontal, non branching lines less than 2 cm long, commonly found in the lower zone periphery, perpendicular to pleural surface. These lines are the thickened, edematous interlobular septa. Causes of Kerley B lines include; pulmonary edema, lymphangitis carcinomatosa and malignant lymphoma, viral and mycoplasmal pneumonia, interstital pulmonary fibrosis, pneumoconiosis, sarcoidosis. These are an evanescent sign on the CXR of a patient in and out of heart failure. The most common cause of Kerley B lines is pulmonary odema.

Kerley Lines A Lines

1–2 mm non-branching lines radiating from the hilum, 2–6 cm long thickened deep, interlobular septa.

Causes of Kerley Lines

- Pulmonary edema
- Infections (viral, mycoplasma)
- Mitral valve disease
- Interstitial pulmonary fibrosis
- Congenital heart disease
- Alveolar cell carcinoma
- Pulmonary venous occlusive disease
- Lymphoma idiopathic (in the elderly)
- Pneumoconiosis
- Lymphangiectasia

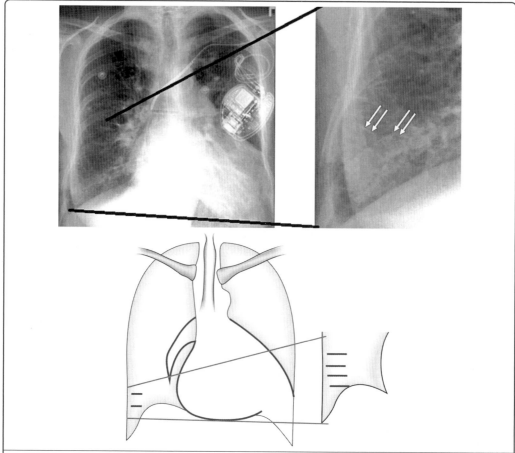

Fig. 3.27: Chest X-ray showing typical Kerley B lines. *Note*: The parallel transverse lines (arrow) perpendicular to pleural surface. The Kerley B lines are due to left ventricular failure in this case

- Lymphangitis carcinomatosis
- Lymphatic obstruction
- Sarcoidosis
- Lymphangiomyomatosis
- Pulmonary hemorrhage

Congestive Cardiac Failure—Pulmonary Edema

There are two basic types of pulmonary edema. One is cardogenic edema caused by increased hydrostatic pulmonary capillary pressure. The other is termed noncardogenic pulmonary edema, and is caused by either altered capillary membrane permeability or decreased plasma oncotic pressure.

On a CXR, cardiogenic pulmonary edema show- cephalization of the pulmonary vessels, Kerley B lines or septal lines, peribronchial cuffing, "batwing" pattern, patchy shadowing with air bronchograms, and increased cardiac size. Unilateral, miliary and lobar or lower zone edema are considered atypical patterns of cardiac pulmonary edema. A unilateral pattern may be caused by lying preferentially on one side. Unusual patterns of edema may be found in patients with chronic obstructive pulmonary disease (COPD) who have predominant upper lobe emphysema.

Most common cause of the pulmonary edema pattern is cardiogenic failure. Usually associated with cardiomegaly (especially if the result of left ventricular failure); other cardiogenic causes include mitral valvular disease, left atrial myxoma, and the hypoplastic left heart syndromes. Noncardiogenic causes include disorders of the pulmonary veins (primary or secondary to mediastinal fibrosis or tumor), veno-occlusive disease, drowning and anomalous pulmonary venous return. Unilateral pulmonary edema is probably most frequently related to dependency. A patchy, asymmetric pattern may develop in patients with emphysema.

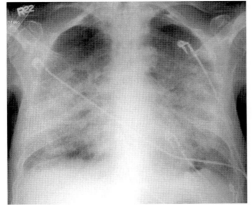 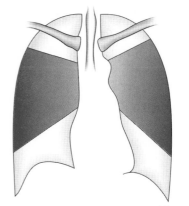

| Chest X-ray showing butterfly wing shaped pulmonary odema in a case of drowning. The opacity is in mid zone, bilateral with air bronchogram. | Note the normal sized heart with no evidence of pulmonary hypertension. |

Fig. 3.28: Chest X-ray showing typical batwing opacity in pulmonary edema

LUNG LUCENCY

❑ LUNG LUCENCY—UNILATERAL INVOLVING WHOLE LUNG

Pneumothorax

A pneumothorax is defined as air inside the pleural cavity.

A spontaneous pneumothorax (PTX) is one that occurs with normal lungs underneath. Most pneumothoraces are iatrogenic and caused by a physician during surgery or central line placement. Trauma, such as a motor vehicle accident is another important cause.

A tension PTX is a type of PTX in which air enters the pleural cavity and is trapped during expiration usually by some type of ball valve-like mechanism. This leads to a buildup of air increasing intrathoracic pressure. Eventually the pressure buildup is large enough to make the lung collapse and shift the mediastinum away from the tension side.

Findings in Chest X-ray in Tension Pneumothorax (Fig. 3.29)

Note the marked density difference between the left and right thoracic cavities. The complete translucency on the left with absence of vascular markings is characteristic of a pneumothorax. What appears as a left hilar mass is in fact the collapsed left lung (passive collapse) retracted into a small central density. The patient is incidentally a female whose breast shadows account for the change in density between the upper and lower lung fields.

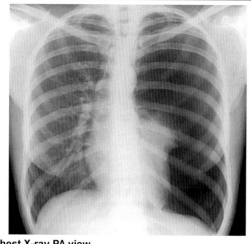

Chest X-ray PA view
Left side tension pneumothorax
Signs of push to right
Trachea and mediastinum are pushed to right side
Note the density difference between two sides, right side normal, left side hyperlucent

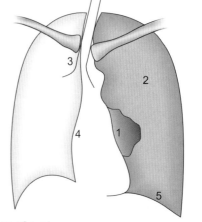

Signs of push
1. Collapsed left lung
2. Air under tension in left pleural cavity
   No bronchovascular markings
3. Tracheal shift to right side
4. Mediastinal shift to right side
Tension pneumothorax left side

Fig. 3.29: Chest X-ray showing tension pneumothorax

❑ LUNG LUCENCY—UNILATERAL INVOLVING PART OF LUNG

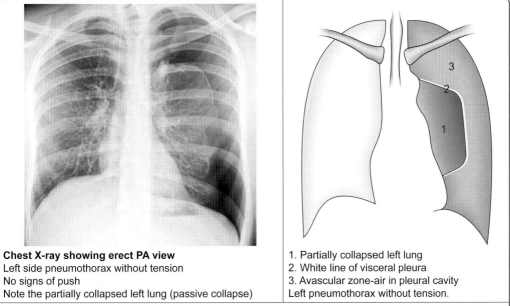

Chest X-ray showing erect PA view Left side pneumothorax without tension No signs of push Note the partially collapsed left lung (passive collapse)	1. Partially collapsed left lung 2. White line of visceral pleura 3. Avascular zone-air in pleural cavity Left pneumothorax without tension.

Fig. 3.30: Chest X-ray showing small pneumothorax

Pneumothorax if it continues, it can compromise venous filling of the heart and even cause death. On chest X-ray, a pneumothorax appears as air without lung markings in the least dependant part of the chest. Generally, the air is found peripheral to the white line of the pleura. In an upright film this is most likely seen in the apices. A small PTX is best demonstrated by an expiration film. It can be difficult to see when the patient is in a supine position. In this position, air rises to the medial aspect of the lung and may be seen as a lucency along the mediastinum. It may also collect in the inferior costophrenic sulci causing a deep sulcus sign.

Radiological Appearances

- With the patient upright, pneumothorax typically appears as a crescent-shape radiolucent area, outlined medially by the sharp white line of the visceral pleura in the upper hemithorax in the affected side, parallel to chest wall with no other vascular marking.
- However, in the supine patient, gas preferentially collects in the antigravity-non-dependent portion of the pleural space, anteromedialy and inferiorly. Consequently, the radiographic findings of pneumothorax in supine X-rays are different from those seen on upright radiographs.

   The radiographic features of pneumothorax on the supine radiograph include the deep sulcus sign (prominence of the costophrenic sulcus) basilar hyperlucency, adjacent to the diaphragm. Unusual sharp delineation of the mediastinal or cardiac contour, and clear visualization of the apical pericardial fat pad.

- Tension pneumothorax is one of the most common life-threatening intrathoracic injures caused by blunt trauma. The diagnosis in most cases is made from clinical signs and symptoms.

  Radiographic findings suggestive of tension pneumothorax include increased lucency of the affected hemithorax with contralateral displacement of the mediastinum and trachea and flattening or even inversion of the ipsilateral hemidiaphragm.

  The size of the pneumothorax (i.e. the volume of air in the pleural space) can be determined with a reasonable degree of accuracy by measuring the distance between the chest wall and the lung. This is relevant to treatment, as smaller pneumothoraces may be managed differently. An air rim of 2 cm means that the pneumothorax occupies about 50% of the hemithorax.

  Deep sulcus sign is useful in confirming suspected pneumothorax on AP supine radiography in compromised patients, such as those in the intensive care setting.

Causes of Unilateral Hyperlucency

- Pneumothorax
- Swyer-James syndrome
- Agenesis of pulmonary artery
- Unilateral partial airway obstruction of large airway

  But the most common cause is pneumothorax.

Deep sulcus sign-This sign refers to a deep collection of intrapleural air (pneumothorax) in the costophrenic sulcus as seen on the supine chest radiograph (Fig. 3.31).

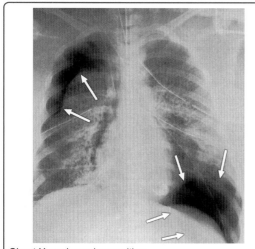 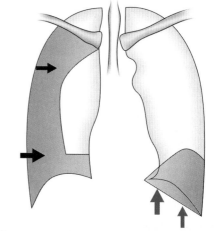

| Chest X-ray in supine position
Note the sharp outline of costophrenic angle and basilar hyperlucency suggesting air collection. | Blue arrows show the deep sulcus sign. Black arrows show the pneumothorax |

Fig. 3.31: Chest X-ray showing deep sulcus sign

A hydropneumothorax is both air and fluid in the pleural space. It is characterized by an air-fluid level on an upright or decubitus film in a patient with a pneumothorax. Some causes of a hydropneumothorax are trauma, thoracentesis, surgery, ruptured esophagus, and empyema. Most important cause is iatrogenic—improper drainage of pleural effusion.

Fibrous-Cavernous Tuberculosis

The most common cause of cavity in our part of the country is pulmonary tuberculosis. The pulmonary tuberculosis in adults characteristically involve the upper lobe. The fibrosis is the hallmark of adult tuberculosis. The lung parenchyma is irreversibly damaged and replaced by fibrosis. The loss of lung volume is proportional to the degree of fibrosis. The presence of cavity indicates that the diseases is in active stage. Further the cavity may be the fore runner of hemoptysis. The cavity is usually thin walled. But due to recurrent infection, superadded other bacterial infection the wall may become thicker. The presence of fungal ball indicates chronicity of the disease. Fibrosis and cavitation can occur simultaneously and form the classical fibrous-cavernous tuberculosis. Fibrosis and cavitation do not occur in children. Atypical tuberculosis manifestations may be seen in immunecompromised patients, eg. HIV.

Lung Abscess

'Primary' lung abscess—large solitary abscess without underlying lung disease is usually due to anerobic bacteria.

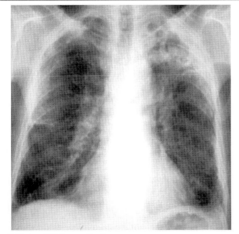

Chest X-ray PA (erect) view
Note a large cavity in left lung upper zone.
The lumen cotains a fungal ball
The walls are thick, irregular
Evidence of fibrosis (signs of pull) in upper lobe is seen
Fibrous-cavernous tuberculosis

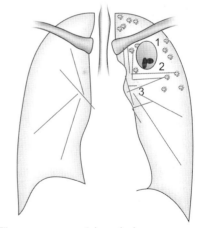

Fibrous cavernous tuberculosis
1. Cavity with a fungal ball
2. Thick walled cavity
3. Fibrotic fibrous-cavernous tuberculosis cstrands showing signs of focal pull
 • left hilum pulled up
 • crowding of ribs

Fig. 3.32: Chest X-ray showing cavitation

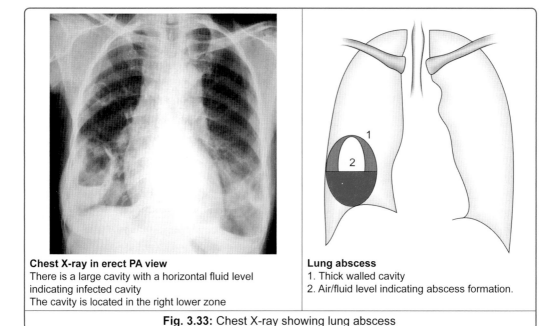

Chest X-ray in erect PA view
There is a large cavity with a horizontal fluid level indicating infected cavity
The cavity is located in the right lower zone

Lung abscess
1. Thick walled cavity
2. Air/fluid level indicating abscess formation.

Fig. 3.33: Chest X-ray showing lung abscess

Secondary lung abscess—a complication of pneumonia, septic emboli, bronchiectasis or associated with aspiration and/or impaired local or systemic immune response (elderly, epileptics, diabetics, alcoholics and the immunosuppressed). Chest X-ray shows a cavitating spherical, usually >2 cm in diameter, but can measure up to 12 cm. There is usually an air-fluid level present, which show fluid shifting. Characteristically the dimensions of the abscess are approximately equal when measured in the frontal and lateral projections. This finding distinguishes a lung abscess from pleural loculated collections.

It is easier to identify if a lung abscess if in centre of lung parenchyma. But if it is located close to chest wall then it is difficult in some cases to differentiate it from empyema (Table 3.8).

Table 3.8 | Empyema vs lung abscess

Empyema	Lung abscess
Lenticular shape	Round shape
Size variable in frontal/lateral views	Size remains same in frontal/lateral views
Surrounding lung compression seen	No Surrounding lung compression
Obtuse angle with chest wall	Acute angle with chest wall
Uniform wall thickness	Non-uniform wall thickness

Pneumatocele

Pulmonary pneumatoceles are thin-walled, air-filled cysts that develop within the lung parenchyma. They can be single emphysematous lesions but are more often multiple, thin-walled, air-filled, cyst like cavities. Most often, they occur as a sequela to acute pneumonia, commonly caused by *Staphylococcus aureus*. Noninfectious etiologies include hydrocarbon ingestion, trauma, and positive pressure ventilation.

Initial chest radiography often reveals pneumonia without evidence of a pneumatocele (FIg. 3.34). Parapneumonic effusion or empyema can be present. Radiographic evidence of a pneumatocele most often occurs on day 5-7 of hospitalization. Rarely, it may be visible on the initial chest radiograph.

In most circumstances, pneumatoceles are asymptomatic and do not require surgical intervention.Treatment of the underlying pneumonia with antibiotics is the first-line therapy. Close observation in the early stages of the infection and periodic follow-up care until resolution of the pneumatocele is usually adequate treatment.

A pneumatocele is a, round thin-walled, air-filled space in the lung. It is most frequently caused by acute pneumonia, trauma, or aspiration of hydrocarbon fluid and is usually transient. The mechanism is believed to be a combination of parenchymal necrosis and check-valve airway obstruction.

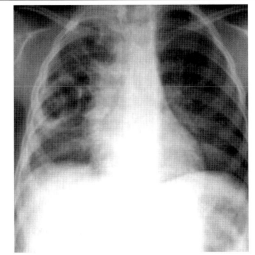

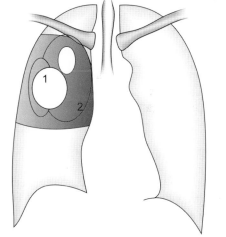

Chest X-ray in a child showing a pneumatocele Multiple cavities, which developed over a period of 24 hours, seen in an area of consolidation. This is typical of staphylococcal pneumonia	1. Multiple thin-walled cavities, of varying sizes, without any fluid level. The cavities developed acutely 2. Surrounding consolidation

Fig. 3.34: Chest X-ray showing pneumatocele

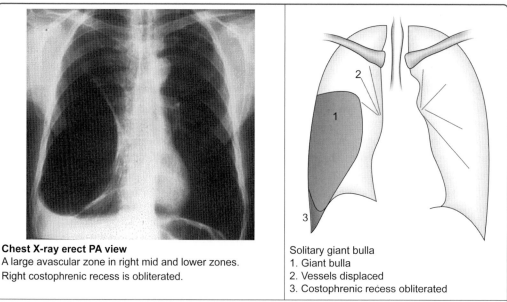

Chest X-ray erect PA view
A large avascular zone in right mid and lower zones.
Right costophrenic recess is obliterated.

Solitary giant bulla
1. Giant bulla
2. Vessels displaced
3. Costophrenic recess obliterated

Fig. 3.35: Chest X-ray showing a bulla

❑ BULLOUS EMPHYSEMA

Bullae are lucent, air-containing spaces that have no vessels and are not perfused. Bullous emphysema is histologically referred to as the presence of emphysematous areas with a complete destruction of lung tissue producing an airspace greater than 1 cm in diameter and with a wall less than 1mm thick. Bullae must be clearly differentiated from other disorders as lung cysts (developmental anomalies; they are lined by respiratory epithelium) and blebs (small sub pleural collections of air). Most of the outer surface of bullae is made of visceral pleura while the inner layer consists of fibrous tissue formed mainly by the destroyed adjacent lung.

❑ BRONCHIECTASIS

Bronchiectasis is defined as permanent abnormal dilatation of bronchi. There is a chronic necrotizing infection of bronchi and bronchioles leading to abnormal permanent dilatation. There is localised irreversible dilatation of bronchi often with thickening of the bronchial wall. The normal bronchial wall should be 'pencil line' thin but in bronchiectasis there is marked wall thickening causing visible, 'tram lines'.

Causes

1. Acquired causes, e.g. bronchial obstruction, due to tumor, foreign bodies and occasionally mucus impaction. Here the lesion is localized to the obstructed lung segment. Post childhood

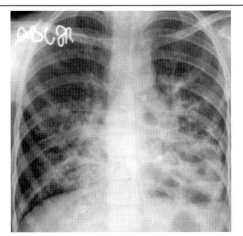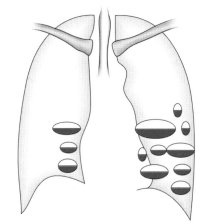

Chest X-ray in erect PA view. Multiple cystic spaces with air-fluid level Involving the entire left lower lobe lingular segment and right middle lobe. Note both the cardiac borders are obscured (silhouette sign) bilateral cystic bronchiectasis secondarily infected.	Bilateral cystic bronchiectasis secondarily infected. Bilateral basal segments cystic bronchiectasis with multiple air-fluid levels within the bronchiectatic cavities.

Fig. 3.36: Chest X-ray showing bronchiectasis

infections (post measles). Diffuse obstruction is commonly seen in chronic bronchitis and atopic asthma tuberculosis, pulmonary fibrosis of any etiology.

2. Congenital or hereditary conditions, e.g. cystic fibrosis, intralobar sequestrations of the lung, immunodeficiency states, immobile cilia, and Kartegener's syndrome. (Bronchiectasis + situs inversus totalis + sinusitis).

Complications of Bronchiectasis

- Hemoptysis, repeated respiratory infection
- Cor pulmonale
- Metastatic abscesses in systemic circulation
- Systemic amyloidosis.

Types of Bronchiectasis

1. Cylindrical or tubular (least severe type)—Bronchi are minimally dilated, have straight regular outlines and end squarely and abruptly.
2. Varicose—Dilation of bronchus with sites of relative construction, bulbous appearance.
3. Saccular or cystic (most severe type)—Ballooned appearance, air/fluid levels.
4. 'Traction bronchiectasis' secondary to pulmonary fibrosis. Is seen in tuberculosis.

Radiological Features

Posterior basal segments of lower lobes most commonly affected.

Bilateral in 50%. Chest X-ray show dilated, thick-walled bronchi giving cystic (bunch of grapes) and tramlining appearance particularly in the lower lobes. Thick-walled bronchus are larger in diameter than accompanying pulmonary artery. In cystic type string or cluster of cysts with discernable walls air/fluid levels within cyst in cylindrical broncheictasis show smooth dilation of bronchus with lack of tapering "tramlines" when seen on plane of scan "Signet ring" when seen in cross section. There may be volume loss and overt 'honeycombing'.

There may be associated areas of infective consolidation and pleuro-parenchymal distortion.

❑ LUNG LUCENCY—BILATERAL COPD

COPD—Emphysema

Emphysema is loss of elastic recoil of the lung with destruction of pulmonary capillary bed and alveolar septa. The end result is air trapping which appears as overinflated lungs and subsequently increased thoracic volume. Emphysema is commonly seen on chest X-ray as diffuse hyperinflation (bilateral symmetrical increased blackiness) with flattening of diaphragms, increased retrosternal space (signs of lung volume increase), bullae (lucent, air-containing spaces that have no vessels) and enlargement of pulmonary artery and right ventricle (secondary to chronic hypoxia) an entity also known as cor pulmonale. Hyperinflation and bullae are the

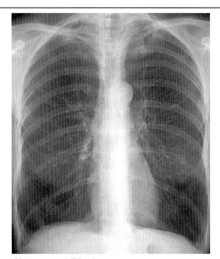

Chest X-ray erect PA view
Bilateral symmetrical hyperlucency.
The domes of diaphragm are at level of posterior 11 rib and anterior 10 rib
Normal dome shape is absent, instead they are flat.
There is increase in thoracic volume-widened intercostals spaces
Senile emphysema COPD

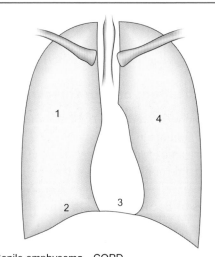

Senile emphysema—COPD
1. Bilateral hyperlucencies
2. Low, flat diaphragm
3. Tubular heart, overdistended lungs
4. Widened intercostal spaces
   (increase in thoracic volume)

Fig. 3.37: Chest X-ray PA view—senile emphysema

best radiographic predictors of emphysema. Barrel shaped chest due to increase in lung volume shown by overinflated lungs, increased retrosternal space, etc.The cardiac shadow may appear small due to overinflated lungs obscuring the true heart borders.This appearance of the heart is called as tubular heart.

However, the radiographic findings correlate poorly with the patient's pulmonary function. Different types of emphysema based on histology are panlobular, intralobular, paraseptal and based on etiology are senile, compensatory, etc.

Emphysema is called an obstructive lung disease because the destruction of lung tissue around smaller sacs, called alveoli, makes these air sacs unable to hold their functional shape upon exhalation. Emphysema is most often caused by tobacco smoking and long-term exposure to air pollution.

In smokers with known emphysema the upper lung zones are commonly more involved than the lower lobes. This situation is reversed in patients with alpha-1 antitrypsin deficiency, where the lower lobes are affected.

Chronic bronchitis commonly occurs in patients with emphysema and is associated with bronchial wall thickening producing the characteristic tramlines.

In compensatory emphysema: When part of the lung is damaged, rest of the lung tissue undergo this type of compensatory emphysema. There is dilation of alveoli not due to destruction of septal walls but compensatory expansion of the residual lung parenchyma after surgical removal of a diseased lung or lobe or collapsed lung segment.

A lateral chest X-ray is necessary to confirm the finding of emphysema seen in frontal projection. In fact the lateral chest X-ray is almost diagnostic of emphysema. The view shows the barrel shaped chest, increased lucency in retrosternal area, low flat diaphragm, increase in

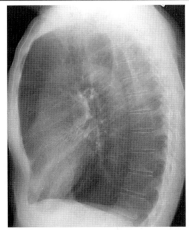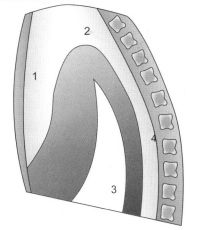

| **Lateral chest X-ray emphysema** Typical barrel shaped chest Increased retrosternal lucency due to emphysema Low flat diaphragm due to air trapping | 1. Increased retrosternal space 2. Diffuse increased lucency 3. Low, flat diaphragm 4. Barrel shaled chest |

Fig. 3.38: Chest X-ray lateral view—senile emphysema

lung volume, overall diffuse lung lucency. Because of air trapping the lung volume remains the same both during inspiration and expiration.

The average annual rate of decline in FEV1 is 20 to 30 mL in normal persons and double that (50 to 60 mL) in smokers with COPD. Smoking cessation delays decline in FEV1 to near normal levels. Stopping smoking is the most effective method to prevent progression of COPD.

Emphysema can be classified into *primary* and *secondary* types. However, it is more commonly classified by location into panacinary and centroacinary (or panacinar and centriacinar, or centrilobular and panlobular).

- *Panacinar* (or *panlobular*) emphysema: The entire respiratory lobule, from respiratory bronchiole to alveoli has expanded. Occurs more commonly in the lower lobes (especially basal segments) and in the anterior margins of the lungs.
- *Centriacinar* (or *centrilobular*) emphysema: The respiratory bronchiole (proximal and central part of the acinus) has expanded. The distal acinus or alveoli are unchanged. It occurs more commonly in the upper lobes.

Diseases of the Heart

Chapter Outline

- ❑ Criteria for a Normal Heart in Chest X-ray
- ❑ Method of Measuring CTR in Chest X-ray
- ❑ How to Read X-ray Chest in Cardiology?
- ❑ Cardiac Shape—A Guide to Congenital Heart Disease
- ❑ Cardiac Situs—A Guide to CHD
- ❑ Coarctation of Aorta
- ❑ PDA
- ❑ Ventricular Septal Defect (VSD)
- ❑ Atrial Septal Defect (ASD)
- ❑ Primary Pulmonary Hypertension

- ❑ Bicuspid Aortic Valve
- ❑ Mitral Regurgitation
- ❑ Rheumatic Mitral Stenosis
- ❑ Left Atrial Enlargement
- ❑ Pericardial Effusion
- ❑ Calcific Pericarditis
- ❑ Dilated Cardiomyopathy
- ❑ Congestive Heart Failure—CHF/CCF
- ❑ Pulmonary Edema
- ❑ Aortic Aneurysm

❑ CRITERIA FOR A NORMAL HEART IN CHEST X-RAY

- Normal CTR is 1:2 (Fig. 4.2), i.e. the width of the heart should be no more than half the width of the chest.
- More than 2/3 to left of midline, less than 1/3 to right of midline, i.e. this normal position is called levocardia (Fig. 4.1).
- The right heart border is formed by the superior vena cava (SVC) above and right atrium below (Fig. 4.3).
- The left heart border is formed from above downwards by aortic knob, pulmonary artery, left auricular appendage and left ventricle (Fig. 4.4).
- The cardiac apex is in left side and is formed by the left ventricle.
- In the pulmonary vasculature of the normal chest, the lower zone pulmonary veins are larger than the upper zone veins due to gravity.

The vena cava are poorly visualized with plain film X-ray, however, the right border of the mediastinum is generally accepted as the right border of the SVC, which should not extend laterally beyond the right border of the heart in a normal individual. The RV is an anterior structure, so it is superimposed on the RA and left ventricle.

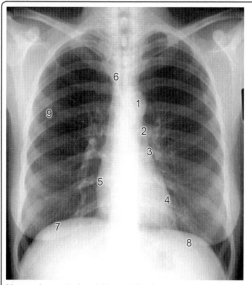
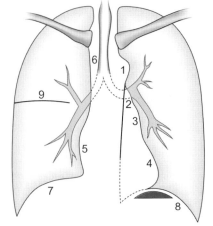

Normal erect chest X-ray PA view
1. Aortic arch
2. Pulmonary trunk
3. Left atrial appendage
4. Left ventricle
5. Right atrium
6. Superior vena cava
7. Right hemidiaphragm
8. Left hemidiaphragm
9. Horizontal fissure

1. Aortic arch
2. Pulmonary trunk
3. Left atrial appendage
4. Left ventricle
5. Right atrium
6. Superior vena cava
7. Right hemidiaphragm
8. Left hemidiaphragm
9. Horizontal fissure

Fig. 4.1: Normal adult chest X-ray showing cardiac structures

Posteroanterior projections of the left heart structures. Ao is the aortic arch, which then continues as the descending aorta, indicated by the dotted line. LAu is the auricle of the left atrium, which itself sits posteriorly at the base of the heart. PV are the pulmonary veins converging on the left atrium. LV is the left ventricle, which is partially posterior to the right ventricle.

❑ METHOD OF MEASURING CTR IN CHEST X-RAY (FIG. 4.2)

A. This is maximum transverse diameter of the heart.
   This is measured between the outermost from the outermost point in right heart border and outermost point in the left heart border.
   Or
   The maximum diameter from midline to outermost part of right side (a) plus the outermost part of left side (b). The sum of (a + b) = A.
B. This is maximum transverse diameter of the thorax.
   This is measured between the inner border of ribs at the level of the diaphragm.
   The ratio of A:B is the CTR.
   Normally, in adults, it is 0.5.

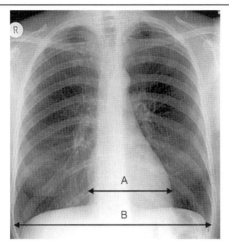

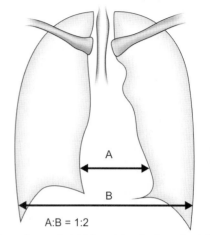

Chest X-ray PA view
A = maximum transverse diameter of the heart
B = maximum transverse diameter of the inner thorax
The ratio A/B must be less than 0.5%

A:B = 1:2

A = outermost right heart border to outer left heart border
B = maximum transverse of thorax measured at the level of diaphragm domes

Fig. 4.2: Method of measuring CTR in chest X-ray

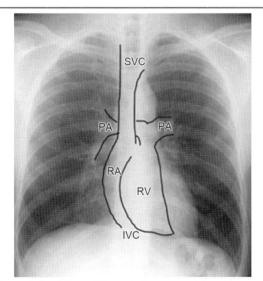

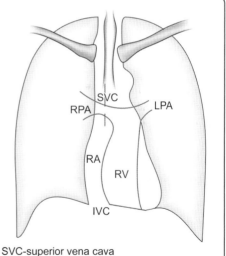

SVC-superior vena cava
RPA-right pulmonary artery
LPA-left pulmonary artery
RA-right atrium
RV-right ventricle
IVC-inferior vena cava
SVC:RA ratio = 1:3

Normal chest X-ray PA erect view
To show-right heart border, position of RA, RV, PA in frontal projection.
Right heart border normally is formed by right atrium and SVC, with contribution by right atrium more than two thirds.

Fig. 4.3: Chest X-ray showing normal right sided cardiac structures

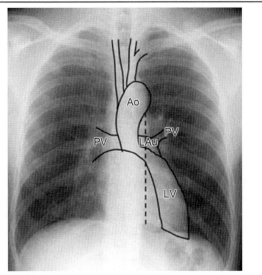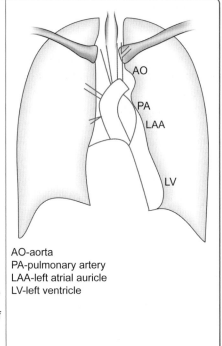

Normal chest X-ray PA, erect view.
Ao-aortic arch, which continues as the descending aorta, indicated by the dotted line.
LAu-auricle of the left atrium, which is posterior at the base of the heart.
PV-pulmonary veins converging on the left atrium.
LV-left ventricle, which is partially posterior to the right ventricle.

AO-aorta
PA-pulmonary artery
LAA-left atrial auricle
LV-left ventricle

Fig. 4.4: Chest X-ray showing normal left sided cardiac structures

Right Sided Cardiac Structures

The right heart border is formed by superior vena cava and right atrium in a normal cardiac situs. The right atrium occupies nearly two-thirds of the border. Further the outermost part of right atrium is less than 2.5 cm from midline. Any enlargement of right atrium may alter these measurements.

Left Sided Cardiac Structures

The left heart border is formed, from above downwards, the aortic knob, pulmonary artery, left auricular appendage and a thin strip of left ventricle in a normal cardiac situs. The apex of the heart is formed by the left ventricle.

An estimate of overall heart size can be made by comparing the maximum width of the cardiac outline with the maximum internal transverse diameter of the thoracic cavity. 'Cardiomegaly' is the term used to describe an enlarged cardiac silhouette where the 'cardiothoracic ratio' is > 0.5. Cardiomegaly is not a sensitive indicator of left ventricular systolic dysfunction since the cardiothoracic ratio is normal in many affected patients.

Dilatation of individual cardiac chambers can be recognised by the characteristic alterations to the cardiac silhouette.

❑ HOW TO READ X-RAY CHEST IN CARDIOLOGY?

Site

We expect the heart shadow to be on the left side. But dextrocardia can occur as evidenced by occupation of major cardiac shadow on the right hemithorax with apex pointing to right. There can be a midline heart also (Mesocardia). Dextrocardia has to be differentiated from dextroposition, where the heart is on the right due to abnormal thoracic structures or changes, e.g. diaphragmatic hernia, agenesis of lung, collapse or fibrosis of lung.

In the presence of true dextrocardia one should make out situs – whether liver is on the right and stomach shadow is on left or vice versa – situs solitus and in versus. In dextrocardia with situs inversus, CHD is present in 5%; in situs solitus with dextrocardia it is 90% and in levocardia with situs in versus CHD occurs in 100%.

Size

Assessment is generally subjective. However, cardiothoracic ratio (CTR) can be measured by measuring maximum internal thoracic diameter at the level of diaphragm and measuring cardiac diameter which is maximum and dividing the latter by former.

Normal CTR in adult is 45% (mean).

Cardiomegaly in adult is CTR ≥ 50%.

In newborn is CTR > 57%.

Infant is CTR > 55%.

A small heart (microcardia) can rarely occur when CTR is less than 40%. It occurs in Addison's disease, anorexia nervosa, severe PEM and in COPD.

Contour

Contour of heart shadow usually gives information regarding ventricular hypertrophy/enlargement.

Mild right ventricular enlargement does not cause cardiomegaly. Modest or marked enlargement causes cardiomegaly with rotated apex which is elevated from diaphragm which gives rise to an upturned apex. An upturned apex without cardiac enlargement occurs in right ventricular hypertrophy.

Left ventricle (LV) is border forming on the left side and hence can be evidently enlarged easily. The apex is shifted down and laterally and even can be below diaphragm. There will be rounding off the apex and elongation of long axis of LV. In DCM heart can be enlarged and can be globular. In LV aneurism, there could be a bulge on left heart border. Cardiomegaly with LV apex occurs in large PDA, VSD, AR, MR and DCM.

Atria

Right atrial enlargement is relatively rare in children. It forms a prominent convexity on the right side which is lower and more lateral. It can be seen as a large diffuse bulge on right side. In adults right atrial enlargement is said to be present if distance from midline to right heart border is > 5.5 cms. In young children it is > 4 cms. RA enlargement can occur in Ebstein, RV EMF and tricuspid atresia.

Left atrial enlargement in frontal view can manifest in many ways.
a. Prominent LA appendage on left border (normally this area is concave)
b. Elevation of left bronchus (well appreciated in well penetrated or digital X-ray)
c. Widening of carinal angle
d. Shadow on shadow (double shadow) appearance.

Great Vessels

Ascending aorta can be border forming on the right side and aortic knuckle is the upper most part of left heart border. Arching – left or right can be made out by ipsilateral indentation of trachea. Dilated aortic shadow can occur in AS, AR, hypertension, coarctation of aorta and aneurism of aorta. Bicuspid aortic valve with no AS can also make aorta prominent.

Main pulmonary artery (MPA) and its branches can be assessed. MPA divides into right and left and the left PA is a continuation of MPA. RPA shortly divides into 2 branches at right hilum – a smaller ascending pulmonary artery and a larger descending pulmonary artery (RDPA). In adults both LPA and descending RPA are between 9 and 15 mm in size near the hilum. Pas are dilated in PS, PAH, idiopathic dilatation, absent pulmonary valve syndrome and in Eisenmenger syndrome.

Pulmonary Vascularity

Abnormal pulmonary vascularity can be generally divided into four types.
1. Oligemia
2. Plethora
3. Pulmonary venous hypertension
4. Pulmonary edema

Pulmonary Oligemia

Vascular shadows are reduced. They are not seen even in the intermediate lung zones. MPA, LPA and right descending PA (RDPA) are all small (Normally RDPA is of the same size as right lower lobe bronchus). Oligemia occurs in TOF, severe PAH, critical PS with reversal of shunt, etc.

Pulmonary Plethora

Vascular shadows are numerous. They are seen in the lateral one third of lung fields. MPA, LPA and RDPA are large. End on vessels are more in number (> 5 in number per both lungs). The end on vessel diameter is more than that of accompanying bronchus. There will be left atrial or right atrial enlargement usually.

Plethora occurs in L → R shunts, admixture lesions and d-TGA without PS. To have plethora L → R should be at least 1.5:1.

Occasionally there can be unilateral plethora as in BT shunt, unilateral MAPCA. Asymmetry in lung vascularity can also occur in Glenn surgery and PA branch stenosis.

Pulmonary Venous Hypertension (PVH)

Normally upper lobe veins are less prominent than lower lobe veins. In PVH there is equalization of the vascularity. When pulmonary venous pressure is > 12 mm Hg, upper lobe veins are equal in size to lower lobe veins. When it is > 15 mm Hg, Kerley B lines (lateral, septal lines) and Kerley A lines (longer, linear lines reaching hilum) are present with occasional pleural effusion. When the pressure is > 25 mm Hg, frank alveolar edema occurs.

Pulmonary Edema

Occurs when pulmonary venous pressure exceeds 25–28 mm Hg. There is alveolar edema, reaching to hilum and a typical 'batwing' appearance.

PVH and edema occur in mitral valve disease, obstructed TAPVC, HLHS, DCM, etc.

Pulmonary vascularity distribution types are shown in Table 4.1.

Table 4.1 | Types of pulmonary vascularity

Type	Example
1. Cephalization	Pulmonary venous HT
2. Centralization (pruning)	Pulmonary venous occlusive disease
3. Lateralization	Unilateral pulmonary embolism
4. Localization	Pulmonary AV fistula
5. Collateralization	Coarctation of aorta, TOG

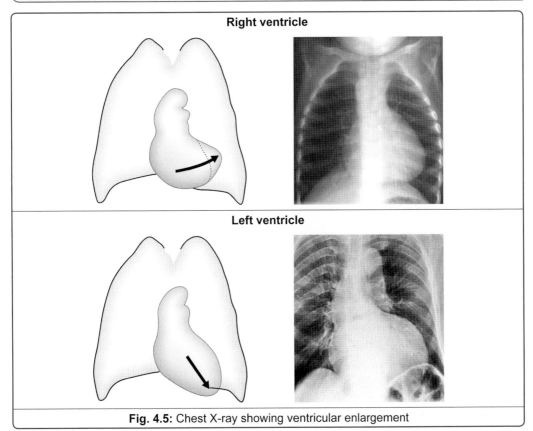

Right ventricle

Left ventricle

Fig. 4.5: Chest X-ray showing ventricular enlargement

Table 4.2 | Quick guide to individual cardiac chamber enlargement

Individual chamber	Specific chamber	Criteria for enlargement (In addition to increased CTR in all)
Right atrium (RA)		1. Right heart border more than 3 cm from midline 2. RA more than 1/3 of RHB
Right ventricle		Cardiac apex is tilted out and upwards. counterclockwise rotation of heart
Left atrium (LA)		1. Dilated LA appendage 2. Widened carinal angle 3. Elevated left main bronchus 4. Double density along, right heart border
Left ventricle		Cardiac apex is tilted out and downwards

Other Abnormalities

They include cervical rib, rib notching (3rd to 8th ribs), ductal calcium, mitral and aortic valve calcium, calcification of aorta, LV aneurism and pericardium, associated pneumonia, collapse and bronchiectasis.

Table 4.3 | Common causes cardiac chamber enlargement

Chamber	Volume overload	Pressure overload
Right atrium	1. Tricuspid regurgitation 2. ASD 3. Pulmonary hypertension 4. T/PAPVD	1. Right ventricular failure 2. Tricuspid stenosis 3. Restrictive CMP 4. Right atrial myxoma
Left atrium	1. Mitral regurgitation 2. VSD 3. PDA 4. ASD with shunt reversal	1. Mitral stenosis 2. Hypertension 3. HOCM 4. LVF 5. Left atrial myxoma
Right ventricle	1. Secondary to LHF, e.g. MVD 2. TR 3. PR	1. Pulmonary arterial hypertension 2. Corpulmonale 3. PS
Left ventricle	MR VSD PDA High cardiac output states Any cause of myocardial damage	Aortic stenosis, systemic hypertension coarctation of the aorta

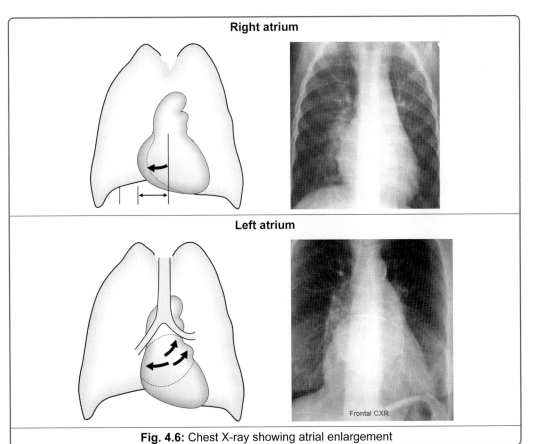

Fig. 4.6: Chest X-ray showing atrial enlargement

Table 4.4 | Quick guide to congenital heart diseases

Acyanotic		Cyanotic	
Increased pulmonary circulation	Normal pulmonary circulation	Increased pulmonary circulation	Normal pulmonary circulation
ASD	PS	TAPVD	TOF
VSD	AS	TA-Type I-III	TAIV
PDA	COA	TGV	TGV
			TA
			Ebstein's anomaly

RA + RV + MPA + PA = ASD
LA + LV + MPA + PA = PDA
LV + RV + MPA = VSD
LA + PVHT + SECO.PAHT + RV = MS
LV + LA + PVHT + SECONDARY PATHOGEN + RV = MS + MR
LV + ASCENDING AORTA = AS
LV + ASCENDING, ARCH AND DESCENDING AORTA = AR
RA + RV = PS, PR

❑ CARDIAC SHAPE—A GUIDE TO CONGENITAL HEART DISEASE

Total Anomalous Pulmonary Venous Drainage (TAPVD)

Pulmonary fields with increased blood flow and prominent pulmonary artery arch are characteristic in this patient.

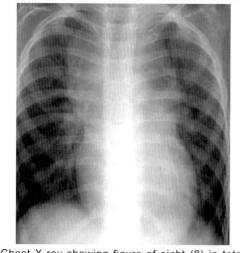

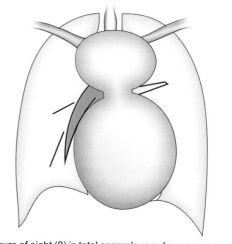

Chest X-ray showing figure of eight (8) in total anomalous pulmonary venous drainage.	Figure of eight (8) in total anomalous pulmonary venous drainage.

Fig. 4.7: Chest X-ray showing typical figure of eight appearance in TAPVD

Right ventricular hypertrophy more easily visualized in lateral projections is almost constant.

Figure of eight or Snowman contour is seen if persistent left superior vena cava is present and is relatively common.

Picture of pulmonary edema with lungs granular appearance is not unusual in the category of patients with pulmonary hypertension and severe heart failure. In the cases where CHF appears during the first month of life the heart size is near normal.

Fallot's Tetralogy

The main features are enlargement of the right ventricle (though overall cardiac size is often normal), decreased pulmonary vascularity, flat or concave pulmonary outflow tract, right aortic arch in approximately 25% of patients. The characteristic features of Fallot's tetralogy are (Fig. 4.8):

1. High ventricular septal defect
2. Obstruction to right ventricular outflow (usually infundibular pulmonary stenosis)
3. Overriding of the aortic orifice above the ventricular defect
4. Right ventricular hypertrophy.

Most common cause of cyanotic congenital heart disease beyond the immediate neonatal period. If there is severe pulmonary stenosis, blood flow from both ventricles is effectively forced into the aorta, causing pronounced bulging of the ascending aorta and prominence of the aortic knob.

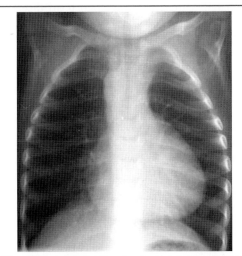 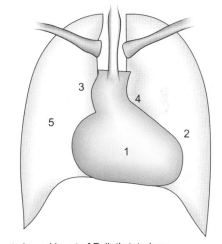

Chest X-ray showing the classical boot shaped heart, concave pulmonary bay due to infundibular pulmonary stenosis and oligemic lung filelds. There is also right sided aortic arch.	Boot shaped heart of Fallot's tetralogy 1. Boot shaped heart 2. Right ventricular hypertrophy 3. Right sided aortic arch 4. Pulmonary bay-flat due to infundibular pulmonary stenosis 5. Pulmonary oligemia

Fig. 4.8: Chest X-ray showing typical boot shape in Fallot's tetralogy

The cardiac silhouette in the AP projection shows "coer in cabot" features due to the lack of pulmonary arch and elevation of the heart apex.

In the lateral view, there is approximation of the cardiac shadow to the thorax anterior wall due to right ventricular hypertrophy.

Lung fields indicate normal or diminished blood flow depending on the degree of pulmonic stenosis. Sometimes increased collateral vasculature can be seen.

Ebstein's Anomaly

Enlargement of the right atrium causes a characteristic squared or boxed appearance of the heart. Decreased pulmonary vascularity; flat or concave pulmonary outflow tract; narrow vascular pedicle and small aortic arch are the main features.

Downward displacement of an incompetent tricuspid valve into the right ventricle so that the upper portion of the right ventricle is effectively incorporated into the right atrium. Functional obstruction to right atrial emptying produces increased pressure and a right-to-left atrial shunt (usually through a patent foramen ovale).

The chest X-ray usually shows a marked globulose cardiomegaly with significant right atrial enlargement (Giant right atrium). If pulmonary stenosis and right to left shunt is present, the lung blood flow will be diminished. The cardiac dynamic is feeble at fluoroscopic examination.

Dextrocardia

In this condition the cardiac apex is in right side of the chest. The aortic arch is in left side. This may be an isolated event or it may be associated with other congenital heart diseases.

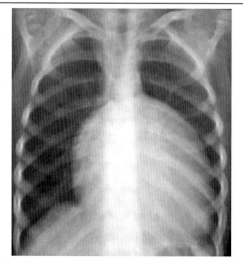 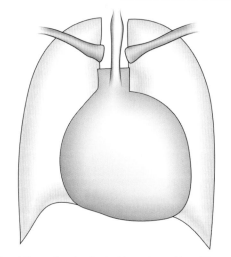

| Chest X-ray showing typical box shaped heart, due to right atrial enlargement. Note the oligemic lung fields. A case of Ebstein's anomaly | Chest X-ray showing typical box shaped heart in case of Ebstein's anomaly |

Fig. 4.9: Chest X-ray showing box shaped heart in Ebstein's anomaly

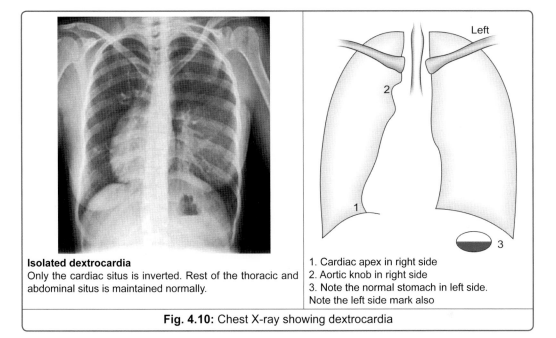

Isolated dextrocardia
Only the cardiac situs is inverted. Rest of the thoracic and abdominal situs is maintained normally.

1. Cardiac apex in right side
2. Aortic knob in right side
3. Note the normal stomach in left side. Note the left side mark also

Fig. 4.10: Chest X-ray showing dextrocardia

Dextrocardia is a congenital defect in which the heart is situated on the right side of the body. There are two main types of dextrocardia: dextrocardia of embryonic arrest (also known as isolated dextrocardia and dextrocardia situs inversus). Dextrocardia is a cardiac positional anomaly in which the heart is located in the right hemithorax with its base-to-apex axis directed to the right and caudad. The malposition is intrinsic to the heart and not caused by extracardiac abnormalities. Dextrocardia should be differentiated from cardiac dextroposition, which is defined as displacement of the heart to the right secondary to extracardiac causes such as right lung hypoplasia, right pneumonectomy, or diaphragmatic hernia. The abdominal situs remains normal, i.e. situs solitus is maintained.

❏ CARDIAC SITUS—A GUIDE TO CHD

Kartagener Syndrome

Characteristics
- Rare syndrome associated with cilia dysmotility.
- Affects respiratory, auditory and sperm cilia.
- Triad of features.
- Situs inversus (50%).
- Nasal polyposis and chronic sinusitis.
- Bronchiectasis.
- Associated with deafness, infertility and other congenital anomalies (e.g. cardiac).
- Familial predisposition.

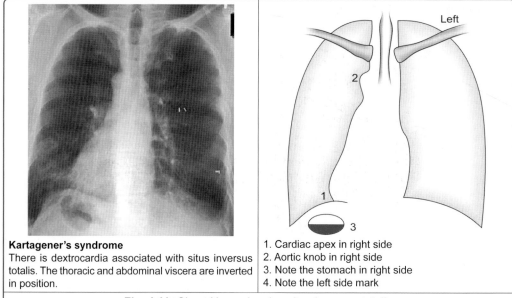

Kartagener's syndrome
There is dextrocardia associated with situs inversus totalis. The thoracic and abdominal viscera are inverted in position.

1. Cardiac apex in right side
2. Aortic knob in right side
3. Note the stomach in right side
4. Note the left side mark

Fig. 4.11: Chest X-ray showing situs inversus totalis

Clinical Features

- Diagnosis in childhood. May be antenatal diagnosis.
- Dyspnea, cough and sputum.
- Recurrent chest infections.

Radiological Features

- CXR—dextrocardiasitus inversus. Bibasal bronchiectasis. May be mucus plugging and lobar collapse or associated infective consolidation.
- Facial X-ray or CT—demonstrates extensive sinus soft tissue in keeping with polyps and mucus.

Differential Diagnosis

- Cystic fibrosis and asthma may have similar appearances particularly as 50% of Kartagener's cases have no dextrocardia.

❑ COARCTATION OF AORTA

Coarctation of the aorta is a stenosis in the aortic arch usually at, or beyond, the site of the ductus venosus. In neonates this is often a sling of ductal tissue that causes narrowing of the lumen when the patent ductus arteriosus closes. In adults there is often a more definite obstruction with luminal narrowing distal to the left subclavian artery.

Congenital narrowing at the junction of the aortic arch and the descending aorta due to a fibrous ridge. More common in males—about 80%.incidence.50% of patients have other

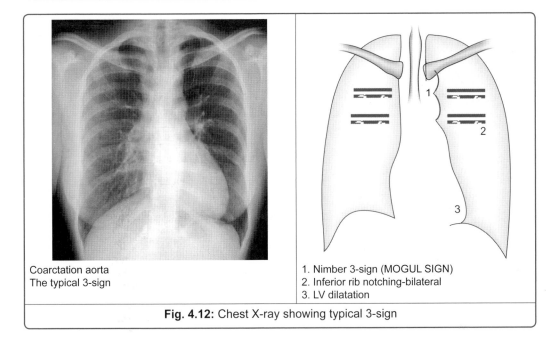

Coarctation aorta
The typical 3-sign

1. Nimber 3-sign (MOGUL SIGN)
2. Inferior rib notching-bilateral
3. LV dilatation

Fig. 4.12: Chest X-ray showing typical 3-sign

radiologically detectable other congenital anomalies like-cerebral berry aneurysm. Bicuspid aortic valve, Turner's syndrome, PDA, VSD, etc.

In adults the characteristic 3-sign caused by pre and post stenotic aortic dilatation in chest X-ray. Further bilateral, symmetrical inferior rib notching is seen in ribs 3–6, due to arterial collaterals supplying blood beyong obstruction. The left ventricle is hypertrophied. The barium swallow shows reverse 3-sign.

In neonates can produce cardiac failure. LVH since early infancy. Many times the LVH diminishes with age due to a larger collateral circulation. There is often a small ascending aorta.

Rib notching (Rossler sign) due to the collateral circulation (more often in 3rd to 8th rib) are seen more often after 4 years of age.

❑ PATENT DUCTUS ARTERIOSUS (PDA)

The ductus arteriosus shunts blood away from the lungs, from the pulmonary artery to the aorta, in utero, and usually closes shortly after birth. If ductal patency persists, there is left to right shunting from the aorta to the pulmonary artery.

The left ventricle increases systolic blood pressure to maintain forward diastolic flow, leading to bounding pulses clinically. The left ventricle and left atrium experience volume overload and dilate, but the right heart does not enlarge unless right ventricular failure develops.

Radiographic findings of PDA include increased pulmonary blood flow, a prominent aortic arch, cardiomegaly, and lung hyperinflation. There may be visualization of the ductus infundibulum in the region of the aortic arch. However, it should be noted that the ductus infundibulum is often seen in normal neonates, but becomes inapparent after the first week of

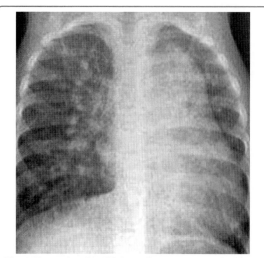
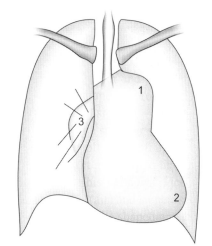

Chest X-ray showing PDA-cardiomegaly grossly dilated pulmonary artery and pulmonary plethora	1. Grossly dilated main pulmonary artery 2. Dilated right pulmonary artery 3. Leftt ventricular enlargement

Fig. 4.13: Chest X-ray showing PDA in failure

life. In long standing PDA, the wall of the ductus infundibulum may become calcified. Later biventricular enlargement is seen.

Roentgenogram Staging

Stage I: The chest X-ray will be normal.
Stage II: Moderate left ventricular hypertrophy. Pulsating enlargment of the aortic knob in contrast with ASD and VSD. Signs of pulmonary plethora.
Stage III: Global cardiomegaly with predominance of the left side. Incipient signs of pulmonary hypertension. Congested hila.
Stage IV: Eisenmenger syndrome.

❑ VENTRICULAR SEPTAL DEFECT (VSD)

The ventricular septum is composed of a muscular septum that can be divided into three major components (inlet, trabecular and outlet) and a small membranous septum lying just underneath the aortic valve.

Ventricular septal defects (VSDs) are classified into three main categories according to their location and margins.

Ventricular septal defects are one of the most common congenital malformations of the heart, accounting for approximately 20% of all congenital cardiac malformations.

A restrictive VSD is defined as a defect which produces a significant pressure gradient between the left ventricle and the right ventricle, is usually accompanied by a small (<1.5/1.0) shunt and does not cause significant hemodynamic derangement.

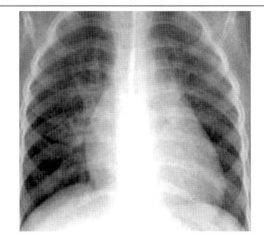 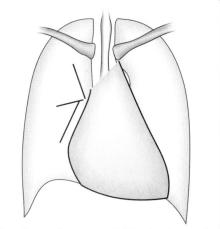

Chest X-ray showing
Left entricular enlargement and increased pulmonary vasculature. Grade II ventricular septal defect.

Line diagram in a case of VSD, showing cardio-megaly and increased pulmonary vasculature.

Fig. 4.14: Chest X-ray showing VSD

Spontaneous closure of a perimembranous VSD or of a small muscular VSD during childhood is common. This is often called Maladie de Roger. Children are most often asymptomatic.

The chest radiograph reflects the magnitude of the shunt as well as the degree of pulmonary hypertension. A moderate sized shunt causes signs of left ventricular dilatation with some pulmonary plethora.

❑ ATRIAL SEPTAL DEFECT (ASD)

One of the most common congenital heart disease (CHD) defects as an isolated lesion, occurring in about 6–10% of all cardiac malformations, presenting in adulthood. ASD and a bicuspid aortic valve are the two most common CHD defects presenting in adulthood. An atrial septal defect (ASD) is a direct communication between the cavities of the atrial chambers, which permits shunting of blood. Secundum ASDs—defects of the oval fossa—are by far the most common. The size of the ASD and the relative compliance of the right ventricle and the pulmonary vascular bed (in relationship to the left ventricle) determine the degree of intra-atrial shunting. Moderate right ventricular hypertrophy more easily appreciated in lateral view with clockwise heart rotation on the longitudinal axis.

Enlargement of pulmonary artery arch to the degree of aneurysm.

Right atrium enlargement, more easily appreciated in lateral or oblique views.

The aorta frequently is smaller than normal.

The left atrium is normal in size.

Dilated hilar vessels. Clear peripheral lung fields with tremendous enlargement of the pulmonary artery and marked hilar congestion will characterize the roentgenogram of severe pulmonary hypertension (more than 60 mm Hg).

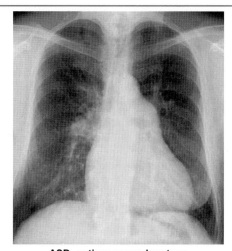
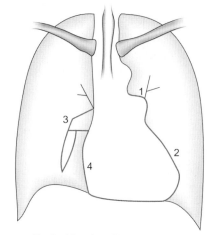

ASD—ostium secundum type	**Typical jug-handle-appearance**
Chest X-ray adult female	1. Groosly dilated pulmonary artery
Classical signs of ASD are seen.	2. Right ventricular dilatation
Typical jug-handle-appearance—handle of jug formed by	3. Dilated right descending pulmonary artery
dilated right pulmonary artery and body of jug formed by	4. Right atrial enlargement
dilated RA and RV due to volume overload.	

Fig. 4.15: Chest X-ray showing atrial septal defect (ASD)

The four types of ASD—ostium primum, ostium secondum, patent foramen ovale, sinus venosus type. Only the secundum is most common.

❑ PRIMARY PULMONARY HYPERTENSION

Primary pulmonary hypertension is an idiopathic disease of young women. The roentgenogram will demonstrate:

- Dilatation of the main pulmonary artery, right and left branches
- Prominent hilar vessels, rapid tapering of the pulmonary vasculature ('peripheral pruning'). Clear peripheral lung fields
- Right ventricular hypertrophy which is better observed in lateral view

  Look for underlying causes, e.g. chronic airways disease, AVMs or heart disease.

In any event, there are no typical signs to differentiate essential pulmonary hypertension from any other kind of systemic pulmonary hypertension, as for example, Eisenmenger's syndrome.

Therefore the diagnosis of primary pulmonary hypertension is by ruling out other causes of pulmonary arterial hypertension.

Pulmonary arterial hypertension is sustained pulmonary arterial pressure >25 mm Hg either due to excessive pulmonary blood flow, e.g. left to right shunts, AVMs and thyrotoxicosis. or obliteration of pulmonary vasculature, e.g. pulmonary arterial emboli, idiopathic (primary pulmonary hypertension), vasculitis and chronic lung disease.

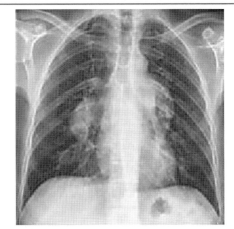

Primary pulmonary arterial hypertension

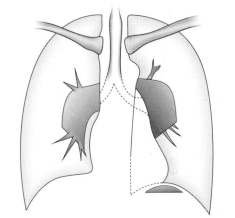

Enlarged central pulmonary arteries. A frontal radiograph in a patient with severe pulmonary arterial hypertension shows markedly enlarged central pulmonary arteries. Note the smooth contours of the arteries.

Fig. 4.16: Chest X-ray showing primary pulmonary hypertension

Differential Diagnosis

The main differential lies within diagnosing the cause of the pulmonary artery enlargement.

Bilateral hilar lymphadenopathy may mimic the CXR appearances of pulmonary arterial hypertension.

❑ BICUSPID AORTIC VALVE

Aortic Stenosis

Calcific Aortic Stenosis

The changes in the natural history of valve disease not only refer to rheumatic heart disease but also to the aortic valve. Previously, aortic stenosis in adults was most commonly due to calcification on a congenitally deformed bicuspid valve. This condition occurs in patients over 30 years old, especially men. The predominant cause of aortic stenosis in western industrialized countries now appears to be degenerative calcific disease in middle-aged or elderly patients. Unlike in mitral stenosis, where calcium is deposited on an already stenosed valve, calcific aortic stenosis results from the deposition of masses of calcium on the aortic cusps which obstruct outflow by their bulk as well as by stiffening the cusps. Thus, calcification *causes* the stenosis. Other common causes include rheumatic heart disease and degeneration of a normal trileaflet aortic valve (usually in a more elderly population).

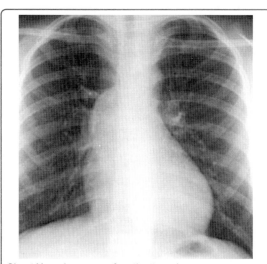

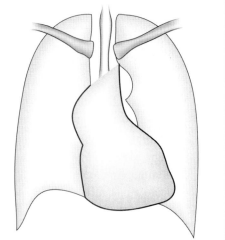

| Chest X-ray in a case of aortic stenosis. Note the LV hypertrophy, dilated ascending aorta (post-stenotic). Normal lung zones. | Line diagram showing isolated left ventricular enlargement. Note the selective dilatation of ascending aorta alone. |

Fig. 4.17: Chest X-ray showing aortic stenosis

Chest Radiography

Rounding of the cardiac apex may suggest left ventricular hypertrophy; however, there is usually some degree of cardiac dilatation, which may be marked if there is aortic regurgitation. Localized prominence of the ascending aorta may indicate post-stenotic dilatation, but in older patients the whole thoracic aorta may be widened from atherosclerosis. The lateral view may show aortic valve calcification. This is best seen by fluoroscopy or CT. The extent of calcification has only a rough relationship to the severity of the stenosis.

Usually the left ventricular hypertrophy, even in severe aortic stenosis, is many times insignificant from the radiological viewpoint. Only in the terminal stages when congestive failure develops and dilatation of the previously reported concentric hypertrophy occurs, the left ventricular shadow will enlarge. Post-stenotic dilatation of the ascending aorta can be seen. In many young children, this aortic dilatation is one of the few radiological findings and in general, its magnitude increases with age. Calcification of the aortic valve is a sign worth looking for, since it is unusual in early age in AS of different etiology (RHD). The analysis of the pulmonic arch is important since the combination of aortic and pulmonic stenosis is not uncommon and it should be excluded before any surgery is considered.

Aortic Regurgitation

Aortic insufficiency (AI), also known as aortic regurgitation (AR), is the leaking of the aortic valve of the heart that causes blood to flow in the reverse direction during ventricular diastole, from the aorta into the left ventricle.

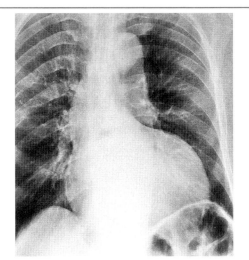 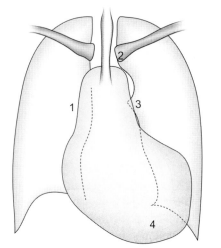

Aortic regurgitation
Chest X-ray showing rounded cardiac apex due to left ventricular dilatation. There is also dilatation of ascending, arch and descending aorta.

Aortic regurgitation
1, 2, 3 are dilated aortic root, arch and descending aorta respectively.
4 LV dilatation. Note the cardiac apex is shifted downwards and below the level of left diaphragmatic dome.

Fig. 4.18: Chest X-ray showing aortic regurgitation

The chest X-ray classically shows marked left ventricular dilatation due to volume overload and dilatation of entire aorta—ascending, arch and descending, unlike aortic stenosis.

Aortic insufficiency can be due to abnormalities of either the aortic valve or the aortic root (the beginning of the aorta). In acute AI, as may be seen with acute perforation of the aortic valve due to endocarditis.

Causes of Aortic Regurgitation in Mneumonics

SCREAM—Aortic regurgitation!
- Syphilis
- Congenital
- Rheumatic fever
- Endocarditis
- Aortic dissection
- Marfan's syndrome
- Ankylosing spondylitis
- Rheumatoid arthriti

❏ MITRAL REGURGITATION

Pulmonary blood flow redistribution is indicated by a decrease in the size and/or number of visible pulmonary vessels in one or more lung regions (with a corresponding increase in number

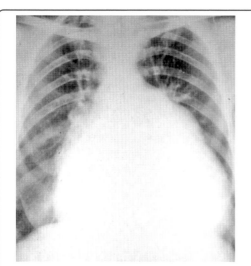 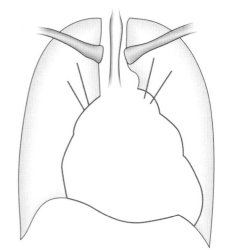

Chest X-ray showing generalized cardiomegaly, especially left ventricular dilatation, left atrium and right atrium. Note also the cephalization of pulmonary blood flow.	Line diagram in a case of mitral regurgitation, showing left ventricular dilatation, gross left atrial enlargement and moderate right atrial enlargement. Note the cephalization of pulmonary venous hypertension.

Fig. 4.19: Chest X-ray showing mitral regurgitation

and/or size of pulmonary vessels in other parts of the lung. Upper lobe blood diversion in patients with mitral valve disease is the archetypal example of redistribution. The degree of left atrial enlargement is greater than that seen in mitral stenosis. There is left ventricular enlargement due to volume overload. Gross left atrial enlargement, dilated left ventricle and signs of venous hypertension are the classical chest X-ray finding in mitral regurgitation. There are several causes of mitral regurgitation and each depicts its abnormality in addition to above findings. The appearances on chest radiography depend on the duration and severity of the mitral regurgitation and any other associated heart disease. Acute, severe, nonrheumatic mitral regurgitation may present with pulmonary edema, but with a virtually normal heart size and shape.

❑ RHEUMATIC MITRAL STENOSIS

This is most common cause of acquired heart disease of the four cardiac valves mitral valve is the most commonly affected. The chest X-ray hallmark of mitral stenosis is left atrial enlargement. The X-ray signs of left atrial enlargement are:

- Widened carinal angle (Fig. 4.21)
- Enlarged left atrial appendage.
- Double density along right heart border.

The above mentioned signs are well shown in the given example.

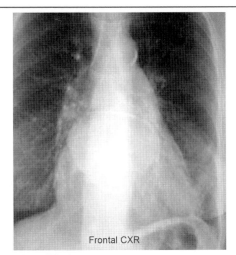

Frontal CXR

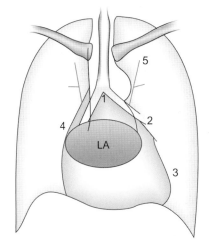

X-ray chest PA view
1. Straight left heart border.
2. Left atrial dilatation.
3. Right atrial and ventricular dilatation.

Rheumatic mitral stenosis
1. Widened carinal angle
2. Enlarged left atrial appendage.
3. Straight left heart border.
4. Double density along right heart border.
1, 2, 4, are signs of left atrial enlargement.

Fig. 4.20: Chest X-ray showing mitral stenosis

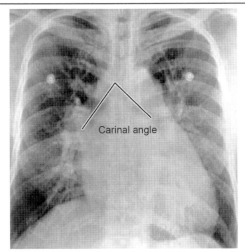

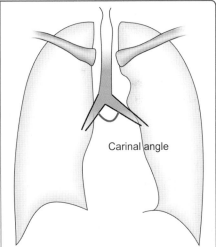

Chest X-ray to show how the carinal angle is measured. Normally it is acute. In cases of left atrial enlargement it becomes obtuse. In this case it is 100 degrees.

The carina is the angle between the tracheal bifurcation into right and left main bronchi.

Fig. 4.21: Chest X-ray to widening of carinal angle in LAE

Apart from left atrial enlargement there is also the classical straight left heart border.

The straight left heart border is due to small aorta, dilated pulmonary artery and left auricular appendage and right ventricular enlargement.

Enlargement of the right ventricle (also the pulmonary outflow tract and central pulmonary arteries) reflects pulmonary arterial hypertension from transmitted increased pressure in the left atrium and the pulmonary veins.

Initially upper lobe vessels are dilated (cephalisation of blood flow), followed by signs of pulmonary venous hypertension and secondary pulmonary artrial hypertension develop.

❑ LEFT ATRIAL ENLARGEMENT

This is the hallmark of mitral stenosis of any etiology. The degree of left atrial enlargement is directly proportional to the degree of mitral stenosis. In mitral stenosis the left atrial enlargement is due to pressure overload. If the degree of left atrial enlargement is gross then there is associated mitral regurgitation is also present. Because of the volume overload the left atrium enlarges to gigantic proportions in mitral regurgitation. Widened carina is the best evidence of left atrial enlargement. Enlarged left atrial appendage, straight left border, double density along the right heart border are some of the other signs of left atrial enlargement.

❑ PERICARDIAL EFFUSION

Pericardial effusion is an abnormal accumulation of fluid in the pericardial cavity. A pericardial effusion with enough pressure to adversely affect heart function is called *cardiac tamponade.*

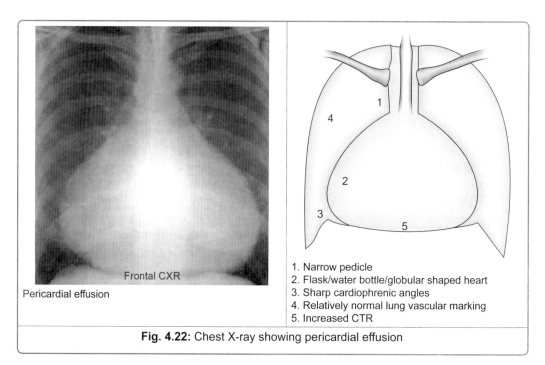

Frontal CXR

Pericardial effusion

1. Narrow pedicle
2. Flask/water bottle/globular shaped heart
3. Sharp cardiophrenic angles
4. Relatively normal lung vascular marking
5. Increased CTR

Fig. 4.22: Chest X-ray showing pericardial effusion

Pericardial effusion usually results from a disturbed equilibrium between the production and re-absorption of pericardial fluid, or from a structural abnormality that allows fluid to enter the pericardial cavity.

Pericardial effusion causes an enlarged heart shadow that is often globular shaped (transverse diameter is disproportionately increased).The increase in cardiac size , unusually sharp cardio-phrenic angles, relatively normal pulmonary vasculature are the main features in chest X-ray.

A "fat pad" sign, a soft tissue stripe wider than 2 mm between the epicardial fat and the anterior mediastinal fat can be seen anterior to the heart on a lateral view.

Approximately 400–500 mL of fluid must be in the pericardium to lead to a detectable change in the size of the heart shadow on PA CXR. It can be critical to diagnose pericardial effusion because if it is acute it may lead to cardiac tamponade, and poor cardiac filling. In the postoperative patient it could be a sign of bleeding.

Asymptomatic effusions are typically first detected by radiography performed for other reasons. A minimum of about 250 mL of fluid collection is required for detection through radiography that augments the cardiac silhouette. Increased pericardial fluid can be hydropericardium (transudate), true pericardial effusion (exudates), pyopericardium (if purulent), hemopericardium (in presence of blood), or mixtures of the above.

❏ CALCIFIC PERICARDITIS

Pericalcification of the pericardium usually is preceded by a prior episode of pericarditis or trauma. Occasionally, pericardial tumors, such as intrapericardial teratomas and pericardial cysts, can calcify.

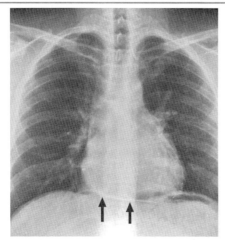 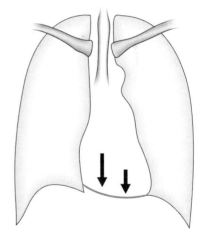

Chest X-ray PA erect shows dense white lines along diaphragmatic pericardial surface, shown by black arrows, suggestive of calcific pericarditis. Note the small heart size and normal pulmonary vasculature.

Line diagram in a case of calcific pericarditis. The gray line indicates site of pericardial calcification.

Fig. 4.23: Chest X-ray showing calcific pericarditis

On chest radiographs, pericardial calcification appears as curvilinear calcification usually affecting the right side of the heart. This is often visualized better on lateral chest radiographs than on frontal views. Calcifications associated with tuberculous pericarditis present as thick, amorphous calcifications along the atrioventricular groove. This pattern may be observed less commonly with other forms of pericarditis as well.

Causes of Pericarditis in Mnemonic

CARDIAC RIND
- Collagen vascular disease, e.g. SLE
- Autoimmune/Aortic aneurysm
- Radiation
- Drugs
- Infection
    - Viral – adenovirus, herpes simplex virus, cytomegalovirus
    - Bacterial – tuberculosis, other bacteria
- Acute renal failure
- Cardiac infarction
- Rheumatic fever
- Injury/Idiopathic
- Neoplasm
- Dressler's syndrome

❑ DILATED CARDIOMYOPATHY

Also known as congestive cardiomyopathy (CCM), dilated cardiomyopathy (DCM) is the most common type of cardiomyopathy. There is global impairment of contractility with dilatation of all chambers, particularly the left ventricle, presenting clinically as congestive cardiac failure. Sometimes symptoms may be noticed after an acute influenza-like illness, hinting that a myocarditis may have been the underlying cause. Chest pain is very unusual. There is a familial form. The plain chest radiograph is almost always abnormal at clinical presentation and most often the only abnormality is cardiac enlargement. The configuration of the heart may be solely left ventricular, or all chambers may be enlarged, although there is usually left ventricular prominence. In the untreated patient, upper lobe blood diversion and a variable degree of pulmonary edema are usually seen. A good response to treatment is indicated by clearing of the pulmonary edema and a reduction of the heart size.

Mneumonic for Dilated Hearts (Extrinsic Heart Diseases)

Dilated Hearts End In Terrible Infiltration
- Dietary – beri-beri (thiamine deficiency)
- Hereditary – familial DCM, muscular dystrophies (Duchenne, myotonia, mitochondrial)
- Endocrine – hypothyroidism, thyrotoxicosis, pheochromocytoma

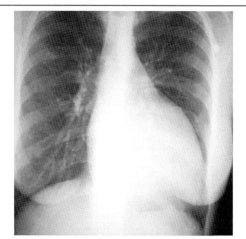 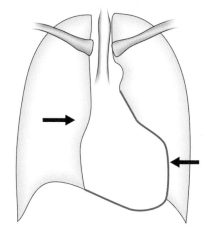

Chest X-ray shows gross left ventricular dilatation with almost normal pulmonary vasculature.	Lower black arrow points to the gross left ventricular dilatation. Upper black arrow points to relatively normal right heart border.

Fig. 4.24: Chest X-ray showing dilated cardiomyopathy

- Infective – viruses (coxsackie), Chagas' disease
- Toxins – alcohol, drugs (anthracyclines)
- Infiltrative – sarcoid, iron overload (hemochromatosis, excess blood transfusions)

☐ CONGESTIVE HEART FAILURE—CHF/CCF

In CCF both sides of heart have failed. CHF may progress to pulmonary venous hypertension and pulmonary edema with leakage of fluid into the interstitium, alveoli and pleural space.

1. The earliest CXR finding of CHF is cardiomegaly, detected as an increased cardiothoracic ratio (>50%).
2. Upper lobe blood diversion. The pulmonary veins running from the upper lobes seem more prominent than those running from the lower lobes. When the pulmonary capillary wedge pressure rises to the 12–18 mm Hg range the upper zone veins dilate and are equal in size or larger, compared to lower lobe vessels. This is called as cephalization.
3. Peribronchial cuffing, enlarged hila, loss of clear space between heart and hila.
4. Kerley B lines. With increasing PCWP (18–24 mm Hg), interstitial edema occurs with the appearance of these lines. They are tiny horizontal lines from the pleural edge and are typical of fluid overload with fluid collecting in the interstitial space.
5. Further increased PCWP above this level is alveolar edema, often in a classic perihilar batwing pattern of density "Bat's wing" haziness around the hila, bilateral pleural effusions.

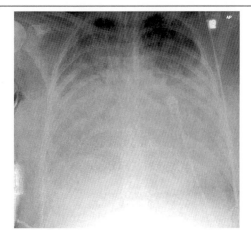 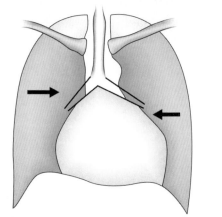

Chest X-ray shows complete white wash due to generalized cardiomegaly and extensive pulmonary edema due to cardiac failure.	Line diagram in a case of cardiogenic pulmonary edema. There is complete white of the lungs due to pulmonary edema. The black arrow points to the bilateral symmetrical hilar enlargement, hilar opacity due to edema.

Fig. 4.25: Chest X-ray showing congestive cardiac failure

6. Alveolar shadowing. In very severe pulmonary edema fluid collects not only in the interstitial space but in the air spaces or alveoli. Hazy shadowing throughout the lungs, and possibly air bronchogram.

Bilateral pleural effusions also often occur. CXR is important in evaluating patients with CHF for development of pulmonary edema and evaluating response to therapy.

❏ PULMONARY EDEMA

Bat's wing distribution describes one of two patterns of consolidation (the other pattern being lobar lung consolidation); refers to the bilateral opacification spreading from the hilar regions into the lungs (sparing the peripheral lung areas) signifying extensive alveolar disease.

The causes of bat's wing are: pulmonary edema in heart failure, fluid overload, hypoproteinemia (Table 4.5).

Heart Failure—Chest X-ray Signs in Mneumonics

ABCDE
- Alveolar edema (Bat's wings), air bronchogram
- kerley B lines (interstitial edema), Bat's wing pattern
- Cardiomegaly, cephalization, increased CTR
- Dilated, prominent upper lobe vessels
- Effusion (pleural)

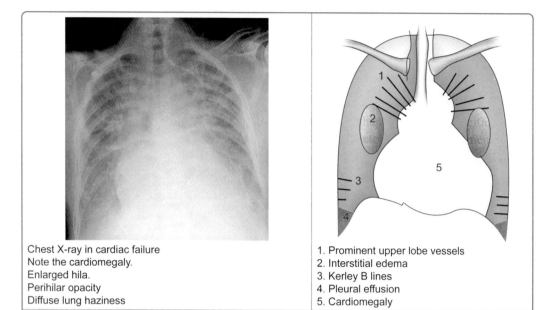

Chest X-ray in cardiac failure
Note the cardiomegaly.
Enlarged hila.
Perihilar opacity
Diffuse lung haziness

1. Prominent upper lobe vessels
2. Interstitial edema
3. Kerley B lines
4. Pleural effusion
5. Cardiomegaly

Fig. 4.26: Chest X-ray showing "batswing" appearance in pulmonary edema

Table 4.5	Causes of pulmonary venous hypertension and pulmonary edema

Left ventricular outflow obstruction, e.g. aortic coarctation, aortic stenosis, hypoplastic left heart
Left ventricular failure
Mitral valve disease
Left atrial myxoma
Fibrosing mediastinitis
Pulmonary veno-occlusive disease

❏ AORTIC ANEURYSM

Permanent localized dilatation of the thoracic aorta. The average diameter of the normal thoracic aorta is <4.5 cm. This is the commonest mediastinal vascular abnormality. Most are fusiform dilatations (some are saccular), associated with degenerative atherosclerosis.

Chest X-ray; a soft tissue mediastinal mass in the region of the aorta, measuring 4–10 cm. Wide tortuous aorta >4.5 cm. Curvilinear calcifications outlining the aortic wall. Left pleural effusions, left apical cap or left lower lobe collapse.

Aneurysm—Causes in Mneumonic

ATTIC
- Atheroma
- Trauma

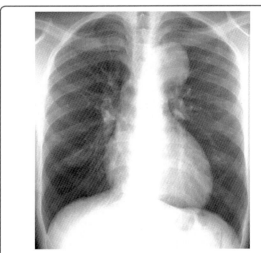

| Chest X-ray PA view showing grossly dilated arch of aorta extending to aortic knob. The CTR is normal. | 1. Saccular aortic aneurysm, arising from aortic knob. |

Fig. 4.27: Chest X-ray showing aortic aneurysm

- Takayasu's aortitis (inflammation)
- Infection, e.g. mycotic aneurysm in endocarditis, syphilis
- Connective tissue disorders, e.g. Marfan's syndrome, Ehlers-Danlos syndrome.

Miscellaneous Lesions

Chapter Outline

❑ Rib Fracture
❑ Cervical Rib
❑ Complete Eventration of the Right Hemidiaphragm
❑ Diaphragm Rupture

❑ Diaphragmatic Hernia in a Child
❑ Gas Under Diaphragm
❑ Chilaiditi Syndrome

❑ RIB FRACTURE (FIG. 5.1)

It is the most common lesion found in ribs.

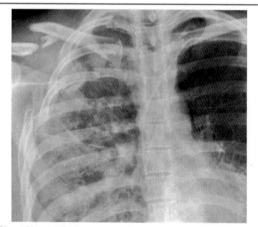

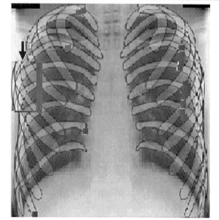

Chest X-ray AP view
Fracture involving the right clavicle and lateral aspect of 5, 6 ribs

Black arrow points to fracture right 5, 6 ribs.

Fig. 5.1: Chest X-ray showing rib fractures

Rib fractures have the appearance of an abrupt discontinuity in the smooth outline of the rib. A lucent fracture line may be seen. Usually chest X-ray is taken to look for fractures in AP projection. For assessing the lower ribs an AP bucky film is required. Since the most important complication of fracture rib is pneumothorax, a routine PA view may be taken. If it is necessary to exclude a rib fracture, oblique rib detail films should be obtained. A common pattern for evaluating the ribs is to examine the posterior portions of the ribs first, then the anterior portions, and finish be examining the lateral aspects of each rib. If you see an abnormality, follow that rib in its entirety. Fracture of the upper three ribs is associated with an increased risk of aortic injury because of the excessive force needed to fracture these ribs. Fracture of the lower three ribs can be associated with liver or spleen injury. Multiple bilateral rib fractures in various stages of healing are associated with child abuse in children or alcohol abuse.

Rib fractures are the most common injury following blunt chest trauma. The most common site of rib fractures are the lateral aspect of ribs 4–9 where there is less overlying musculature. However, fracture of the first and/or second rib is a marker of high energy trauma since these ribs are short, thick, and relatively well-protected by the thoracic muscles. Injuries associated with first and second rib fractures include pulmonary, aortic and cardiac contusion, neck injuries, and severe abdominal injuries. Isolated first rib fractures are also associated with whiplash injuries. Lacerations of the liver, spleen, and kidney are associated with fractures of ribs 9–12. While a common injury, not all rib fractures are identified on the initial chest radiograph, particularly when they are not displaced. Flail chest deformity is a serious manifestation of ribfracture and is defined as 5 or more adjacent rib fractures or more than 3 segmental rib fractures. Flail chest deformity can lead to respiratory failure from the direct effect of lung and pleural injury as well as impaired ventilation due to dysfunction of normal chest wall mechanics.

❑ CERVICAL RIB

A cervical rib (Fig. 5.2) is a supernumerary (or extra) rib which arises from the seventh cervical vertebra. Their presence is a congenital abnormality located above the normal first rib. A cervical rib is present in only about 1 in 500 (0.2%) of people, even rarer cases, an individual may have two cervical ribs. In some persons, it may be bilateral. Usually a complete rib may be formed. But sometimes it may be incomplete.

The presence of a cervical rib can cause a form of thoracic outlet syndrome due to compression of the lower trunk of the brachial plexus or subclavian artery. These structures are entrapped between the cervical rib and scalenus muscle.

❑ COMPLETE EVENTRATION OF THE RIGHT HEMIDIAPHRAGM (FIG. 5.3)

Eventration is unilateral hypoplasia of a hemidiaphragm (very rarely both) with the thinned, weakened musculature inadequate to restrain the abdominal viscera. Localized eventration primarily involves the anteromedial portion of the right hemidiaphragm, through which a portion of the right lobe of the liver bulges. In a posterior eventration, upward displacement of the kidney can produce a rounded mass. Total eventration occurs almost exclusively on the left. Eventrations may have paradoxical diaphragmatic motion (though more commonly seen

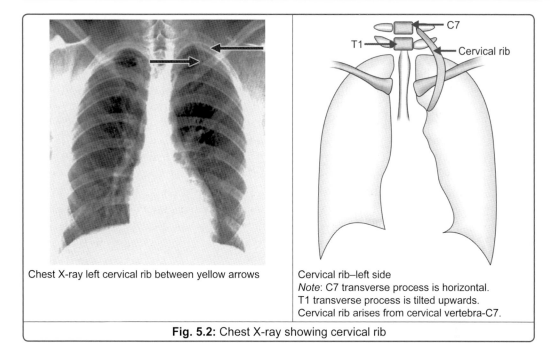

| Chest X-ray left cervical rib between yellow arrows | Cervical rib—left side
Note: C7 transverse process is horizontal.
T1 transverse process is tilted upwards.
Cervical rib arises from cervical vertebra-C7. |

Fig. 5.2: Chest X-ray showing cervical rib

in diaphragmatic paralysis). There may be a mediastinal shift to opposite. The eventration may involve only part of right dome, wherein only left lobe of liver migrates upwards. This is more common in children.

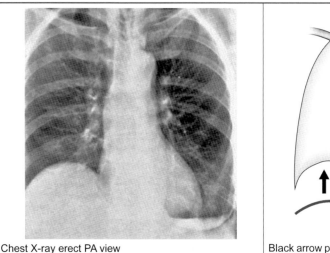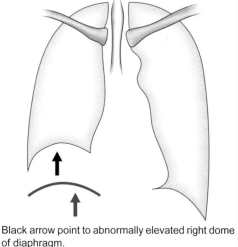

| Chest X-ray erect PA view
Abnormally elevated right dome of diaphragm, indicating eventration. | Black arrow point to abnormally elevated right dome of diaphragm.
Blue line arrow shows the normal expected level. |

Fig. 5.3: Chest X-ray showing eventration of right dome of diaphragm

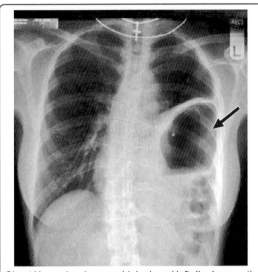

Chest X-ray showing very high placed left diaphragmatic dome.The gas shadows seen below the abnormal left dome are that of herniated stomach and large bowel.

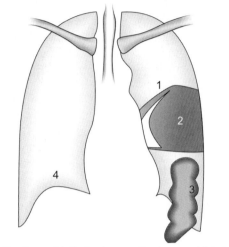

1. Rupture of left diaphragmatic dome, which is highly placed
2. Herniated stomach
3. Herniated large bowel
4. Normal right dome of diaphragm

Fig. 5.4: Chest X-ray showing traumatic rupture of left dome

❏ DIAPHRAGM RUPTURE

Most common in left side, about 90%, There is history of blunt injury only 5% of cases.The presentation is very late after the accident. Initially missed in 70% of cases. Diaphragmatic tears are common and commonly missed. The most common location is the central tendon, extending posterolaterally.

Diaphragmatic hernias are common. It is more common on the left side and is associated with other congenital anomalies. Bochdalek hernias are the most common congenital diaphragmatic hernias and the ratio of left to right sided diaphragmatic defects is approximately 9:1. These hernias are located in the posterolateral portion of the diaphragm. This is thought to be due to the fact that the liver affords protection on the right side. They appear as soft tissue masses arising from the posterior aspect of the hemidiaphragm on the radiograph. Small defects contain fat, larger defects can contain stomach, spleen, kidney, or liver. If small, Bochdalek hernias may remain undetected until later on in life since they are almost always asymptomatic. On a lateral chest film, a single, smooth focal bulge is seen centered approximately 4 to 5 cm anterior to the posterior diaphragmatic insertion.

Morgagni hernias are anteriomedial and more common on the right side. Herniation occurs through the sternal costal area. These hernias are associated with obesity and usually contain fat. The transverse colon herniation are asymptomatic, some may complain of respiratory or epigastric pressure or pain. In the hiatal hernia—the stomach slips through the esophageal hiatus

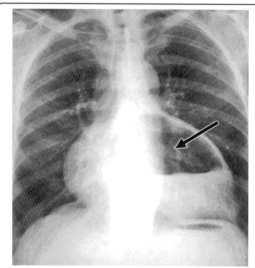 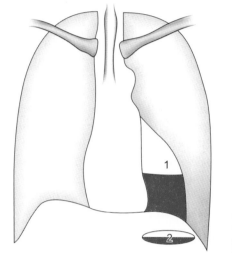

Chest X-ray in erect PA view
A large air-fluid level in left side of posterior mediastinum
A lateral chest X-ray and fluroscopy confirmed it to be a hiatus hernia

1. Air-fluid in posterior mediastinum due to herniated stomach (Hiatus Hernia)
2. Normal air/fluid level in part of stomach

Fig. 5.5: Chest X-ray showing sliding hiatus hernia

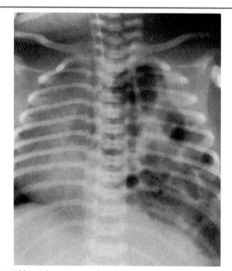 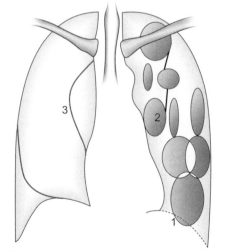

Chest X-ray in a case of diaphragmatic hernia.
Note the bowel loops in left hemithorax, mediastinal shift to right side.

1. Nonvisualization of left dome of diaphragm
2. Multiple round air lucencies suggestive of herniated bowel loops into the thorax
3. Mediastinal shift to right side.

Fig. 5.6: Chest X-ray showing diaphragmatic hernia in a child

into the chest. Weakness of the diaphragm can occur without frank herniation of abdominal contents. This is termed an eventration, and it usually occurs on the right with a portion of the liver bulging cephalad.

❑ DIAPHRAGMATIC HERNIA IN A CHILD

An early chest radiograph is obtained to confirm the diagnosis of congenital diaphragmatic hernia. Findings include loops of bowel in the chest, mediastinal shift, paucity of bowel gas in the abdomen, and presence of the tip of a nasogastric tube in the thoracic stomach (Fig. 5.7). Repeated chest radiography may reveal a change in the intrathoracic gas pattern.

Right-sided lesions are difficult to differentiate from diaphragmatic eventration and lobar consolidation.

The diagnosis of congenital diaphragmatic hernia is frequently made prenatally prior to 25 weeks' gestation.

Congenital diaphragmatic hernia is usually detected in the antenatal period (46–97%), depending on the use of level II ultrasonography techniques. Ultrasonography reveals polyhydramnios, an absent intra-abdominal gastric air bubble, mediastinal shift, and hydrops fetalis. Ultrasonography demonstrates the dynamic nature of the visceral herniation observed with congenital diaphragmatic hernia. The visceral hernia has moved in and out of the chest in several fetuses.

The pathophysiology of congenital diaphragmatic hernia involves pulmonary hypoplasia, pulmonary hypertension, pulmonary immaturity, and potential deficiencies in the surfactant and antioxidant enzyme system.

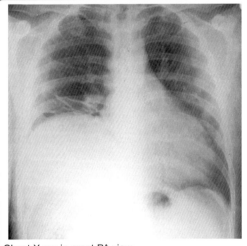

Chest X-ray in erect PA view.
Grossly elevated right dome of diaphragm

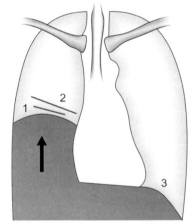

1. Abnormally elevated right dome of diaphragm (black arrow)
2. Right basal lung showing plate atelectasis
3. Normally placed left dome of diaphragm

Fig. 5.7: Chest X-ray showing abnormal elevation of right diaphragmatic dome

Unilateral Elevation of the Hemidiaphragm

It can be seen as a result of an enlargement or displacement of an abdominal organ, a subpulmonic process such as effusion, loss of volume of the lung with lobar atelectasis or surgical resection, or hemidiaphragmatic paralysis. Diaphragmatic paralysis results from interruption of the phrenic nerve supply to the diaphragm. The most common cause is malignancy, such as bronchogenic carcinoma, or postsurgical trauma. Hepatomegaly secondary to amoebic liver abscess is also common.

Other causes of diaphragmatic paralysis include polio, herpes, infections, lead poisoning, pulmonary infarctions, pneumonia, mediastinitis, and pericarditis. The diagnosis of unilateral paralysis of the diaphragm is suggested by the finding of an elevated hemidiaphragm on the chest X-ray. With diaphragmatic paralysis, the negative pleural pressure tends to pull the paralyzed diaphragm upward. Normally the right diaphragm is about 3 cm higher than the left. Confirmation of diaphragmatic paralysis is established by the sniff test. In this test the diaphragm is observed fluoroscopically as the patient sniffs. The normal diaphragm is moved downward during the sniff maneuver as the diaphragmatic muscles contract. A paralyzed diaphragm moves paradoxically upward because of negative pleural pressure. Patients with paralyzed diaphragms may be asymptomatic or may complain of dyspnea on lying down or with exertion. With complete paralysis, vital capacity and total lung capacity may be reduced about 25% from the baseline, and the maximum inspiratory pressure is reduced to about 40%.

❑ GAS UNDER DIAPHRAGM

Gas under right dome of diaphragm (Fig. 5.8) is the classical sign of perforation of an abdominal viscus. An erect abdomen X-ray or a chest would be sufficient to demonstrate gas under the diaphragm.

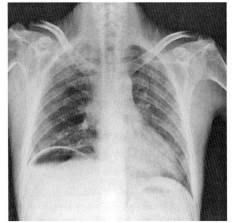 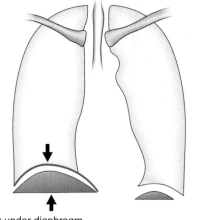

Black air shadow is seen under the white line of the right diaphragmatic dome.	Air under diaphragm Upper arrow–right dome of diaphragm Lower arrow-free air in peritoneal cavity

Fig. 5.8: Chest X-ray showing gas under right dome of diaphragm

Gastrointestinal perforation is a complete penetration of the wall of the stomach, small intestine or large bowel, resulting in intestinal contents flowing into the abdominal cavity. Perforation of the intestines results in the potential for bacterial contamination of the abdominal cavity (a condition known as peritonitis). Perforation of the stomach can lead to a chemical peritonitis due to leaked gastric acid. Perforation anywhere along the gastrointestinal tract is a surgical emergency. Underlying causes include gastric ulcer, appendicitis, gastrointestinal cancer, diverticulitis, superior mesenteric artery syndrome, trauma and ascariasis. Typhoid fever, non-steroidal anti-inflammatory drugs, ingestion of corrosives may also be responsible. In abdominal/decubitus X-ray:

- Locules of gas lying outside bowel often with odd/linear margins.
- Both sides of the bowel may be visible (Rigler's sign).
- The falciform ligament may be demonstrated.
- Hyperlucency overlying the liver with clear inferior hepatic margin outlined by air.

❑ CHILAIDITI SYNDROME

Chilaiditi syndrome (Fig. 5.9) is a rare condition when pain occurs due to transposition of a loop of large intestine (usually transverse colon) in between the diaphragm and the liver, visible on plain abdominal X-ray or chest X-ray. Normally this causes no symptoms, and this is called Chilaiditi's sign. The sign can be permanently present, or sporadically. This anatomical variant is sometimes mistaken for the more serious condition of having air under the diaphragm (pneumoperitoneum) which is usually an indication of bowel perforation, possibly leading to unnecessary surgical interventions. Chilaiditi syndrome refers only to complications in the

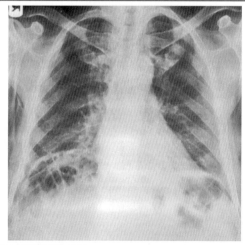
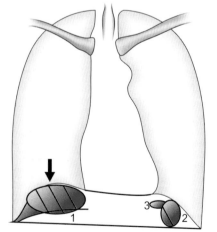

| Chest X-ray PA view Gas under right dome confined within the colon Note the multiple haustrations of colon. | Arrow points to right diaphragmatic dome 1. Abnormal colonic gas shadow 2. Normal colonic gas shadow 3. Normal gastric air bubble |

Fig. 5.9: Chest X-ray showing colon beneath right dome (Chilaiditi syndrome)

presence of Chilaiditi's sign. These include abdominal pain, torsion of the bowel (transverse colon volvulus) or shortness of breath. Differential diagnosis is subphrenic abscess.

The findings in subphrenic abscess are focal walled-off infected intra-abdominal collection lying in the sub-diaphragmatic space. Usually right sided, elevated hemidiaphragm. Pleural effusion (reactive). Subphrenic lucency or air-fluid level.

Subcutaneous Emphysema (Fig. 5.10)

It is also known as surgical emphysema and tissue emphysema, occurs when gas or air is present in the subcutaneous layer of the skin. Subcutaneous refers to the tissue beneath the cutis of the skin, and emphysema refers to trapped air. Since the air generally comes from the chest cavity, subcutaneous emphysema usually occurs on the chest, neck and face, where it is able to travel from the chest cavity along the fascia. Subcutaneous emphysema has a characteristic crackling feel to the touch, subcutaneous emphysema can result from puncture of parts of the respiratory or gastrointestinal systems. Particularly in the chest and neck, air may become trapped as a result of penetrating trauma (e.g. gunshot wounds or stab wounds) or blunt trauma. Infection (e.g. gas gangrene) can cause gas to be trapped in the subcutaneous tissues. Subcutaneous emphysema can be caused by medical procedures and medical conditions that cause the pressure in the alveoli of the lung to be higher than that in the tissues outside of them. Its most common causes are pneumothorax and a chest tube that has become occluded by a blood clot or fibrinous material. It can also occur spontaneously due to rupture of the alveoli with dramatic presentation. When the condition is caused by surgery it is called surgical emphysema.

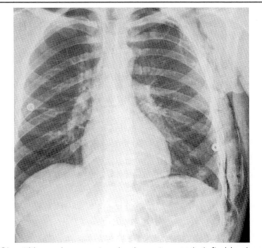

Chest X-ray shows extensive lucent areas in left side chest wall, extending upto axilla. In case of blunt chest injury this suggests subcutaneous emphysema.
Subcutaneous/Surgical emphysema

Line diagram shows black areas, shown by black arrows, within the left side chest wall

Fig. 5.10: Chest X-ray showing subcutaneous emphysema

The Tables 5.1 and 5.2, and figure 5.11 show the common chest tubes/catheters seen in an intensive care chest X-ray.

Table 5.1 | Some chest tubes-position

Tubes	Correct position
1. Endotracheal tube	3–5 cm above the carina
2. Nasogastric tubes	Tip and side holes should be 10 cm into the stomach
3. Central venous line	Tip should be in the superior vena cava, just above the right atrium
4. Swan-Ganz catheter	Tip should be in pulmonary artery and no more than 2–4 cm beyond the vertebral midline
5. Pacemaker	Pacemaker: Look for point of origin, location of wires – transvenous, epicardial, or permanent nerator. Atrial lead should be in the right atrium, ventricular lead in the right ventricle
6. Chest tubes: Location	Inserted high in apex for pneumothorax, low in bases for effusions or hemo-thorax
7. Intra-aortic balloon catheter	Tip should be in the aorta – 2 cm below the aortic arch

Table 5.2 | Some useful chest X-ray signs

Radiographic sign in CXR	Finding/interpretation/example
1. Silhouette sign	Loss of the contour of the heart or diaphragm indicating an adjacent abnormality (e.g. atelectasis of the right middle lobe obscures the right-hand side of the heart's border)
2. Air bronchogram	Indicates airless alveoli and, therefore, a parenchymal process as distinguished from a pleural or mediastinal process
3. Air crescent sign	Indicates solid material in a lung cavity, often due to a fungus ball, or crescentic cavitation in invasive fungal infection
4. Cervicothoracic sign	A mediastinal opacity that projects above the clavicles, situated posterior to the plane of the trachea, while an opacity projecting at or below the clavicles is situated anteriorly
5. Tapered margins	A lesion in the chest wall, mediastinum or pleura may have smooth tapered borders and obtuse angles with the chest wall or mediastinum, while parenchymal lesions usually form acute angles
6. Gloved finger sign	Indicates lobar collapse with a central mass, often due to an obstructing bronchogenic carcinoma in an adult
7. Golden sign	Indicates lobar collapse with a central mass, often due to an obstructing bronchogenic carcinoma in an adult
8. Deep sulcus sign	Indicates pneumothorax on a supine radiograph

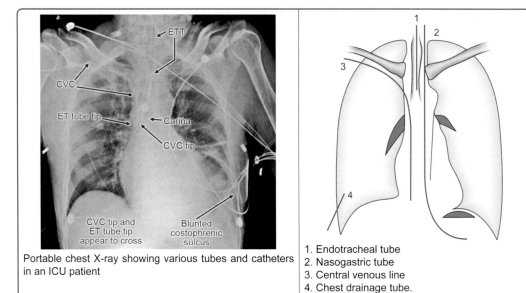

Portable chest X-ray showing various tubes and catheters in an ICU patient

1. Endotracheal tube
2. Nasogastric tube
3. Central venous line
4. Chest drainage tube.

Fig. 5.11: Chest X-ray showing various tubes/catheters

Index

Page numbers followed by 'f' indicate figures

A

ASD   91
Air bronchogram signs   24
Air under diaphragm   111
Aortic
    aneurysm   103
    regurgitation   94
    stenosis   93
Application of silhouette sign   22

B

Basic radiographic
    contrast   10
    density   9
Bilateral hilar lymphadenopathy   58
Boot shaped heart in Fallot's tetralogy   85
Box shaped heart in Ebstein's anomaly   86
Bronchiectasis   70

C

Calcific pericarditis   99
Cardiac chamber
    atrial enlargement   83
    ventricle enlargement   81
Cervical rib   106
Chest lateral   15*f*
Chest tubes/catheters   115*f*
Chilaiditi syndrome   112
Congestive cardiac failure   61, 102*f*
Costophrenic angles   18*f*

D

Deep sulcus sign   66
Depth of respiration   6
Diaphragmatic
    hernia   109*f*
    rupture   108*f*
Dilated cardiomyopathy   100

E

Eventration of diaphragm   106
Extrapleural sign   27

F

Fibrous-cavernous tuberculosis   55*f*, 67
Figure of eight in TAPVD   84*f*

G

Giant bulla   70*f*
Golden's "S" sign   41

H

Hiatus hernia   109*f*

I

Inspiratory/expiratory film   7*f*
Isolated dextrocardia   87*f*

K

Kartagener syndrome   87
Kerley B lines   61

L

Left lung
    central mass   46
    peripheral mass   48
Lobar
    left upper lobe collapse   38*f*
    middle lobe consolidation   35*f*
    upper lobe consolidation   36*f*
    right upper lobe collapse   39*f*
Luftsichel sign   42
Lung
    abscess   67
    cavitation   67*f*

lobes orientation   16*f*
zones   17*f*

M

Massive
    collapse   32
    consolidation   33
    pleural effusion   31
Mediastinal lymphoma   60*f*
Miliary mottling   52
    nodules   52
Mitral
    regurgitation   95
    stenosis   96
Multiple lung secondaries   49

N

Normal
    cardiac silhouette with lung lobes   24*f*
    chest X-ray PA erect   14*f*
    chest X-ray for cardiac structures   19*f*
    CTR measurement   19*f*
    left heart structures   21*f*
    right heart structures   20*f*

P

Pancoast tumor   46
Patient
    positioning   4*f*
    rotation   7
PDA in failure   89, 90*f*

Penetration   5
Pericardial effusion   98
Pleural effusion   45
Pneumatocele   69
Pneumothorax   64
Post-pneumonectomy   34*f*
Primary
    complex   56
    pulmonary hypertension   92
Pulmonary edema
    butterfly's wing pattern   63

R

Rib fracture   105
Rib orientation   18*f*

S

Sarcoidosis   58
Senile lung emphysema
    lateral view   73*f*
    PA view   72*f*
Solitary pulmonary nodule   51*f*
Subcutaneous emphysema   113

T

Tram lines   26
Tuberculoma   51
Typical 3-sign in coarctation of aorta   89*f*

V

VSD   90